# Commitment in Couples Therapy

*Commitment in Couples Therapy* offers a comprehensive clinical guide to help those who work with couples determine the authenticity of a couple's commitment, and to guide their decision on whether the relationship is worth salvaging.

The purpose of this book is to focus on those couples who have joined for reasons that pose a significant chance of relational failure. This specific dyad entails one seemingly "committed" partner and one apparently "less committed" partner, both of whom may be conscious or unconscious about their sabotaging behavior in the relationship. Betchen offers a clinical model to treat the commitment issue and help the couple's therapist skillfully uncover each partner's conflict with commitment, determine the couple's true relational status, and determine how to re-contract the relationship on more authentic grounds. Chapters provide coverage of the unconscious match process, the sociocultural, transactional, familial, and psychological factors behind commitment, and countertransference, with case studies throughout. Finally, this book offers critical assessment and treatment strategies for therapists to implement in their practice.

This book is an essential read for mental health clinicians of all levels, and a valuable resource for graduate students in marriage and family therapy programs.

**Stephen J. Betchen**, DSW, is a licensed marriage and family therapist and a certified sex therapist. He is also an AAMFT Approved Supervisor and AASECT Certified Supervisor. He maintains a private practice in New Jersey specializing in couples and sex therapy.

"Once again, Dr. Betchen masterfully refines his Conflict Theory focusing on the specific area of romantic commitment. In this text, he provides the therapist with a formula for assessing and treating romantic commitment conflicts; thus, alleviating the couple's symptom, and promoting a more durable relationship. *Commitment in Couples Therapy* is an essential read for therapists at any juncture of practice."

**Nancy Gambescia, PhD,** *Former Director, Post-Graduate Sex Therapy Program, Council for Relationships, Philadelphia, Pennsylvania*

"Stephen Betchen has made another significant contribution to the couples therapy literature. His insights into couples' conflict and commitment are certain to enrich the practice of every couples therapist. This is also a must read for those couples experiencing distress and disappointment in their intimate relationship. Betchen's writing style makes this text accessible to all, and his wealth of knowledge and experience promises to improve the lives of both experienced clinicians and distressed couples. After 40+ years of clinical practice, I still learn from the work of Dr. Betchen. This book will have a prominent place on my bookshelf for many years to come."

**Daniel N. Watter, EdD,** *Past-President, The Society for Sex Therapy and Research (SSTAR)*

"Stephen Betchen's latest work is like reading a master therapy chef's favorite couples' cookbook – one in which the key ingredients of the couple's lack of commitment are connected to the couple's shared underlying conflict, which when revealed and treated with Betchen's model, can ultimately lead to a more durable relationship."

**Jay Lappin, MSW,** *Minuchin Center for the Family, New York*

# Commitment in Couples Therapy

A Therapist's Guide to Assessing
Relationship Durability

Stephen J. Betchen

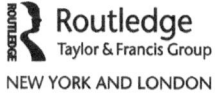

Routledge
Taylor & Francis Group

NEW YORK AND LONDON

Designed cover image: Getty Images

First published 2025
by Routledge
605 Third Avenue, New York, NY 10158

and by Routledge
4 Park Square, Milton Park, Abingdon, Oxon, OX14 4RN

*Routledge is an imprint of the Taylor & Francis Group, an informa business*

© 2025 Stephen J. Betchen

ISBN: 978-1-032-75812-1 (hbk)
ISBN: 978-1-032-75809-1 (pbk)
ISBN: 978-1-003-47574-3 (ebk)

DOI: 10.4324/9781003475743

Typeset in Optima
by codeMantra

To my wife Bonnie, for her inspiration and unwavering support.

# Contents

# About the Author

**Stephen J. Betchen**, DSW, is a licensed marriage and family therapist and a certified sex therapist. He received his doctorate at the University of Pennsylvania with a specialization in marriage and family therapy and trained at the Marriage Council of Philadelphia, Department of Psychiatry, University of Pennsylvania School of Medicine. He then completed a post-doctoral fellowship at the New York Hospital-Cornell University Medical Center in psychology with a specialization in sex therapy-under Helen Singer Kaplan. Subsequently, he was awarded a clinical psychoanalytic fellowship (classical) by the Institute of the Philadelphia Association for Psychoanalysis. He also is a graduate of the Intensive Psychoanalytic Psychotherapy Program (interpersonal/relational) at the William Alanson White Institute and is currently in the Object Relations Theory and Practice Program at the International Psychotherapy Institute. He is the author of approximately 200 scholarly articles and chapters, magazine pieces and blogs, over 500 newspaper columns, and seven books on relationships. He is an AAMFT fellow and approved supervisor and an AASECT diplomate and certified supervisor. He is also a former adjunct clinical professor in the Department of Couple and Family Therapy at Thomas Jefferson University and chief supervisor in the post-graduate Sex Therapy Program at the Council for Relationships. He currently writes a blog on relationships for *PsychologyToday.com* and maintains a full-time private practice specializing in couples/sex therapy in Cherry Hill, New Jersey.

# Acknowledgments

As always, I wish to thank the many couples I have treated over the years, especially those who committed to the arduous task of accumulating personal insight and taking responsibility for their behavior. I also thank my editor, Julia Giordano, for giving me the opportunity to write this book and for making it a pleasurable and productive experience.

# Preface

When I first began studying commitment, I had no idea how complex and pervasive the concept is. There were numerous articles and books on commitment in relation to one's workplace, organization, religion, and social contexts. However, given my area of expertise, I was most interested in what is commonly referred to as "romantic commitment," or the commitment between partners or lovers. Continuing my focus on this specific material, I learned that low commitment is now considered "the" most common reason given for divorce, supplanting infidelity and domestic violence. Certainly, a concept worthy of further clinical study.

This book was born out of many years of treating couples with low commitment and the realization of just how difficult and deflating this process can be. Colleagues have confessed there is nothing more frustrating than attempting to treat a couple with low commitment or one lacking in durability. One couples therapist told me that it gives him a feeling of "clinical hopelessness." A relationship with low romantic commitment may resemble a business or transactional arrangement or be on the verge of ending. Those partners who do manage to stay together with little commitment are usually not symptom free. They may also unconsciously transmit this commitment problem from relationship to relationship with disastrous results.

I also found that couples with low commitment were inadequate and symptomatic in one or more of the following key ingredients of commitment necessary for relationship durability: attachment, love, passion, or intimacy. Not all ingredients need to be present for relationship durability. But if there is not some semblance of each present, the relationship may be vulnerable. The real trouble occurs when partners cannot agree on balancing these ingredients in a way that is comfortable to both. For example, if one partner wants more intimacy and the other does not.

Another finding that caught my attention is that couples lacking in commitment are typically made up of one partner playing the role of the committed partner and the other partner playing the role of the uncommitted. The seemingly committed partner gives no overt indication of a problem with commitment. In fact, this partner continuously pursues the seemingly uncommitted or avoidant partner for greater commitment, usually in any one or more of the key ingredients mentioned. Committed and uncommitted partners each have their own distinct traits and tendencies. For example, the uncommitted may be manipulative, distant, or sadistic. The committed may appear needy and masochistic and have low self-worth. But no matter how different they may look, each plays a complementary role impacting the key ingredients of commitment, thus leading to the couple's symptoms.

Committed and uncommitted partners do not choose a complementary mate by chance. I have found that partners have an unconscious tendency to choose others who, like themselves, have an internal conflict with commitment. And while conflict is a vehicle for attraction, if not balanced between the needs of each partner, it can also produce symptoms in any one of the key ingredients of commitment. I found Robert J. Sternberg's triangular theory especially useful as a reference on this matter.

This conflict is predominately unconscious and referred to as a *committed vs. uncommitted* conflict. That is, each partner has internalized two parts: one part needs the stability and security of commitment, while the other part is uncomfortable with commitment and tends to sabotage it. The partner playing the uncommitted role cannot commit to others, while the partner playing the role of the committed mate cannot allow others to commit to them. And while both partners have the same conflict with commitment, the conflict manifests differently in each depending upon experiences in their respective families of origin.

In sum, while assessing and treating countless couples, I believe that an underlying conflict with commitment may be responsible for a variety of relationship symptoms, which will show in one or more of the concept's key ingredients of love, attachment, intimacy, and passion. If partners are satisfied with the levels of these ingredients or are symptom free, the conflict may still exist but is considered balanced and under control. If, however, they do not agree on the level, they may be symptomatic in that ingredient and others as well. This couple's conflict would then be considered unbalanced or out-of-control.

The purpose of this book is to provide the couples therapist with a guide on how to accurately assess a conflict with romantic commitment in a couple and to balance this conflict in a way that alleviates the couple's symptoms and, in turn, leads to a long-lasting, more durable relationship. A synopsis of the chapters follows.

- Section 1: Understanding Commitment in Couples – in "Chapter 1. Introduction: Definition and Key Ingredients," I offer a definition of romantic commitment and the concept's relationship and interplay with its key ingredients: love, attachment, intimacy, and passion. Further reflections on commitment and its ingredients are provided including the importance of attachment in forming and maintaining a healthy romantic commitment, the risk of commitment when its ingredients are missing or inadequate, commitment and its ingredients on a continuum, and the role development plays in commitment and its ingredients.

- "Chapter 2. Romantic Commitment: Types and Tendencies." When a couple chooses psychotherapy because of problems (symptoms) with one or more of the key ingredients of commitment, one partner plays the role of the committed partner and the other plays the role of the uncommitted partner. The committed partner projects commitment by pursuing or by being a selfless pleaser, for example, whereas the uncommitted partner may present as distant, disengaged, and selfish. Each partner type is examined individually and in combination.

- "Chapter 3. Romantic Commitment and Conflict" suggests that a couple's symptoms are caused by a shared underlying conflict with commitment that also determines mate choice. That is, two partners sharing the same conflict with commitment are unconsciously drawn to each other. After having established a shared conflict, the couple then colludes to maintain it thus preventing deeper change.

- "Chapter 4. The Origin of the Romantic Committed and Uncommitted" examines the origin of a couple's commitment issues to determine how they are transmitted from one generation to the next. Verbal and nonverbal messages that support low commitment, certain behaviors witnessed in the family of origin, and specific family dynamics may all lead to commitment issues in adulthood.

- Section II. Clinical Assessment of Romantic Commitment – in "Chapter 5. Assessing Couples with Commitment Conflicts," I offer an extensive procedure to assess the commitment and durability of a couple. I use the genogram as an assessment tool and present four cases to demonstrate the assessment process.

- Section III. Clinical Treatment of Romantic Commitment – in "Chapter 6. Treating Couples with Commitment Conflicts," I present three cases in full detail. Each case begins with an assessment and demonstrates how to use a step-by-step approach to treat the couple's symptoms and underlying conflict with commitment.

- Section IV. The Therapist's Conflict with Commitment – "Chapter 7. The Therapist's Commitment" examines three key areas that the couples therapist must consider when treating a couple with a conflict with romantic commitment: (1) commitment to the profession (e.g., therapist dedication to and immersion in the profession); (2) commitment to the self (e.g., therapist self-care); and (3) commitment to the couple (e.g., therapist dedication to the couple and treatment process).

# Section I

# Understanding Commitment in Couples

# Chapter 1

# Introduction
## Definition and Key Ingredients

Many agree that *commitment* indicates a dedication to someone or something. Agnew (2009) said: "At its root, commitment can be defined as intending to continue in a line of action" (p. 2). Much of the literature, however, portrays commitment as a far more complex and wide-reaching concept. Michael et al. (2015) referred to commitment as the "cornerstone of human social life" (p. 1). Indeed the concept has been applied to one's job or career (Rusbult & Farrell, 1983; Van der Heijden et al., 2022), organization (Grego-Planer, 2019; Meyer et al., 2002), social network (Jones, 2018; Surra et al., 2012), relationship with family members (Fehr, 2012; Thomas et al., 2017), religion (Aman et al., 2019), and a commitment to certain tasks (Clark, 2006; Michael et al., 2015).

Some scholars categorize the various characteristics and contexts of commitment. For example, Cervini (2023) distinguished between *emotional commitment*, defined as "the type of commitment that stems from deep feelings, attachments, and emotional investments. It is characterized by a strong bond formed between individuals based on trust"; *moral commitment*, "which revolves around adherence to ethical principles, personal values, and a sense of duty"; *structural commitment*, which is "centered around the obligations and responsibilities that arise from various social roles and contracts"; and *time-based commitment*, which entails "dedicating one's time, energy, and resources to achieving long-term goals" (p. 1).

Johnson (2012) separated commitment into *moral commitment*, or "feeling morally obligated to stay"; *personal commitment*, or "the sense of wanting to stay"; and *structural commitment*, which refers to "feeling constrained to stay regardless of the level of one's personal or moral commitments" (p. 74).

DOI: 10.4324/9781003475743-2

## Romantic Commitment

The focus of this book is on *romantic commitment*, used interchangeably with couple's commitment or commitment between partners in romantic relationships. Morgan and Shaver (2012) wrote:

> Although commitment to a career, organization, or a project has many features in common with commitment to a loved one, the latter seems different in its depth and dependence on innate mechanisms. This is indicated in part by the security accompanying committed romantic relationships. Few objects of commitment provide the fundamental sense of love-worthiness and connectedness experienced by people who are securely attached to a loving partner.
>
> (p. 121)

Few in professional literature disagree with Morgan and Shaver (2012). Day et al. (2011) suggested that romantic commitment gives life meaning. And while there is always overlap in defining the concept, scholars stand by their distinct definitions. Rusbult (1983) defined romantic commitment as "the tendency to maintain a relationship and to feel psychologically attached to it" (p. 102). Agnew (2009) said: "relationship commitment may be viewed as intending to continue in a relationship with a given person" (p. 2). Stanley and Markman (1992) described commitment as a "personal dedication to the relationship and constraints against leaving it" (p. 1). And Wiecha (2023) defined commitment as "an umbrella that refers to the behavior and attitude of a person in a romantic relationship. An emotionally involved partner is loyal, attentive, interested, committed, caring, and loving" (p. 595).

When romantic commitment is high in a relationship and partners feel more attached, couples have been found to be less anxious (Morgan & Shaver, 2012), happier, and more satisfied (Londero-Santos et al., 2021); possess a positive self-concept and increased self-esteem (Gómez-López et al., 2019; Rill et al., 2009); are physically healthier (Weir, 2018); and have better sex lives (Seiter, 2023).

When commitment is low, it can lead to contrasting results and even the destruction of the relationship. Studies have found "low commitment," sometimes referred to as high ambivalence, to be the major cause of relationship dissolution (Amato & Hartmann-Marriott, 2007; Bieber & Ramirez, 2024; Schoebi et al., 2012). It has recently overtaken infidelity as the leading cause of divorce (Gillette, 2022; Gold Buscho, 2021; Scott et al., 2013). According to a national survey by the Gitnux Market Data Report, 73% of the participants reported that "lack of commitment" was the main cause of their divorce. This was followed by frequent arguing (56%), infidelity (55%), unmet expectations (45%), lack of preparation for marriage (41%), and domestic violence (25%) (Lindner, 2024).

## Key Ingredients

Sternberg (1998) found that *love* is related to three overlapping yet independent concepts: *commitment, intimacy,* and *passion.* In his triangular theory of love, the author wrote: "You can have any one without either or both of the others" (p. 6). A couple can be intimate and committed without passion or have passion without intimacy or commitment. Couples can also love without passion, intimacy, or commitment. Ainsworth et al. (1978) found that love is related to *attachment.*

I, however, begin with the concept of *romantic commitment* and view it as consisting of four key ingredients: love, attachment, intimacy, and passion. I believe that when a couple present for treatment and are deemed to have a problem with commitment, they are usually suffering from a void or deficiency in one or more of these ingredients. That is, if a couple has commitment issues, they will most likely show symptoms related to one or more of these key ingredients.

The objective of this chapter is not to conduct an exhaustive study of each ingredient. Rather, it is to examine the connection between romantic commitment and its key ingredients and to show how commitment problems are evident in gaps in one or more of these ingredients. Many couples focus on their symptoms (i.e., problems with the ingredients) and neglect the complexity and danger of low commitment in their relationships.

### Love

Kochar and Sharma (2015) stated: "*Love* is a combination of emotions, cognitions, and behaviors that often plays a critical role in intimate romantic relationships" (p. 1). Lovering (2022) defined love as "an emotion of strong affection, tenderness, or devotion toward a subject or object" (p. 1). According to Ackerman et al. (2011), when an individual utters the words "I love you" to another, they are committing to that individual and their relationship. It moves a short-term relationship into a potentially long-term union.

Scholars have also categorized love. Hatfield and Walster (1978) distinguished between *passionate* and *companionate* love. They wrote:

> Passionate love is a wildly emotional state, a confusion of feelings: tenderness and sexuality, elation and pain, anxiety and relief, altruism and jealousy. Companionate love, on the other hand, is a lower-key emotion. It is friendly affection and deep attachment to someone.
>
> (p. 2)

The authors claimed that companionate love is less intense, exhibits tenderness, and takes longer to develop.

Sternberg (2019) also distinguished between types of love. He stated:

Infatuated love results from the experiencing of passion without the simultaneous experiencing of the other components of love. Empty love comes from the decision that one feels love towards another and is committed to the love in the absence of the intimacy and passion components. Romantic love comes from a combination of intimacy and passion. Companionate love comes from a combination of intimacy and decision/commitment. Fatuous love comes from a combination of passion and decision/commitment in the absence of intimacy. Consummate, or complete love, comes from the combination of all three components: intimacy, passion, and commitment.

(p. 282)

Love can be applied to many different contexts. For example, there is love for family and friends and, most germane to commitment, the love between romantic partners, including those of the same sex (Ackerman et al., 2011; Lovering, 2022).

From a biological/chemical perspective, Fisher (2004), in her book *Why We Love,* separated romantic love into three categories, all fueled by hormones stemming from the hypothalamus of the brain: (1) *lust* (testosterone and estrogen) – the desire for sexual gratification, and a need to reproduce. Fisher called lust "a primordial feeling" (p. 79); (2) *attraction* (dopamine and norepinephrine) – doing things that feel good, or reward behavior; and (3) *attachment* (oxytosin vasopressin) – the ability to be intimate and to form long-term relationships. Fisher wrote that with time, excitement, passion, and ecstasy dissipate in a relationship. "But if you are fortunate, this magic transforms itself into new feelings of security, comfort, calm, and union with your partner" (p. 86). She claimed that these feelings create one of attachment.

Evolutionary scientists also support the link between love and commitment. Harrison (2022) asserted: "a declaration of romantic love is a key point in commitment" (p. 402). Buss (2019), an evolutionary psychologist, claimed that love facilitates commitment or "emerges primarily in the context of long-term mating" (p. 59). He also contended that love beckons the commitment of reproductivity, fosters partner exclusivity or mate guarding, and leads to successful reproductive outcomes and greater parental investment in children. And E. O. Wilson (2000), author of *Sociobiology: The New Synthesis*, wrote: "Love joins hate, aggression, fear, expansiveness, withdrawal, and so on; in blends designed not to promote happiness and survival of the individual, but to favor the maximum transmission of the controlling genes" (p. 4). In this vain, Wilson further theorized that most species evolved from polygamy to monogamy for the following three reasons: (1) two adults are needed to share in the defense of their territory; (2) the need for two adults to cope with the environment; and (3) because married pairs "cooperate more smoothly from the beginning of courtship and nesting" and are therefore better able to breed (p. 330).

Some who study love distinguish between *love* and *being in love* in couples (Gillis, 2023; McCoy, 2018). Being in love is considered more intense and likely to occur in the beginning of a romantic relationship when attraction and excitement are at their highest. Loving someone evolves in relationships and is more associated with the desire to be with another or to be attached to them. Loving and being in love overlap at times. For example, while it may be rare, some older couples will claim to be just as in love as they were in the earlier part of their relationships.

While the therapist should strive to determine whether two partners love or are in love with each other, some partners make it easy for them by conveying the message of love in an unenthusiastic, clinical tone, one lacking in sincerity and passion. In this case the odds are that the deliverer of the message may love the other, but it is less likely they are in love with them. In my clinical practice, I have witnessed partners ending a commitment while simultaneously claiming to love their counterpart. The following are a few examples.

Jill had made up her mind to leave her husband Larry of 22 years. Larry begged her to attend couples therapy to try and salvage their relationship, but she agreed only because she was afraid Larry would hurt himself. Jill was looking for a smooth exit from the marriage. When Larry asked Jill if she still loved him, she responded: "Of course I love you, Larry. It is not like I want you to get hit by a truck or something. I just cannot live with you anymore. I am no longer in love with you."

Tina decided to leave her husband, Kirk, and confronted him in couples therapy. Upset, Kirk asked Tina if she still loved him. Tina responded: "I still love you, Kirk. I just do not feel about you the way a wife should feel about her husband." When I asked whether she was in love with Kirk, Tina said: "No, I can't say that I am in love with him."

When asked to specifically describe the differences between loving a partner and being in love, both Jill and Tina claimed that the love they experienced had more to do with feelings of obligation and respect – not necessarily respect for their husbands per se but because they had spent most of their lives with them. Jill made a point to say:

No matter what happens, Larry is still the father of my children and deserves a certain amount of consideration. My children will be in enough pain because of the divorce. I do not need to add to that by being cold to their father or wishing him ill will.

Both Jill and Tina conceptualized being "in love" with feelings of affection, a strong emotional and physical attraction, and a high level of devotion. Jill claimed that when she is in love, she feels as if she has found her soul mate. "I feel no jealousy towards other women even if they are with someone better looking, richer, or more attentive." Tina said that when she is in love with a man, she does not see any other man in the room but him. "My focus is completely on him. I feel as if I will do anything for him. I have an overwhelming feeling of passion for this person as well."

Echoing Tina, when a partner claims to be in love, no matter what their developmental level, I have found there to be a strong attraction and desire for the other. A certain intensity exists in the relationship as well as an air of optimism. There is usually no immediate threat, if any, to end the relationship. Partners who are in love usually seek treatment for lesser offenses such as a misunderstanding, a minor problem, or a communication issue. Consider the following examples.

Calvin and Jazmine, a Black couple in their 50s, were clearly in love and openly claimed that their marriage was not in any jeopardy. While they presented for "a disagreement on how to spend excess cash," it was clear they each held an attraction, both emotionally and physically for each other, and a deep respect for the other's opinion. Neither partner rejected the other's position but had difficulty understanding it. Calvin, for example, wanted to spend the money on a vacation, and Jazmine first wanted to repair their roof before using the money for a trip. Calvin's idea was to limit what he would spend for a vacation and take the leftover money to fix the roof. In this sense, both Calvin and Jazmine wanted the same things, just not in the same order. Given they were in love with each other, they were easily able to negotiate a compromise: Calvin allowed Jasmine to choose the vacation and price so that enough money was left to fix their roof.

Daniel and William were a long-term, monogamous gay couple who were strongly attracted to each other both emotionally and physically. They appeared totally dedicated to each other and close to each other's families. The couple appeared embarrassed to seek treatment, but they reported that their sex life had dwindled in the last several months. Daniel wanted to expand their sexual repertoire but was afraid to tell William. Daniel claimed that William was far more conservative than he, and he was afraid it would frighten him off. William was confused as to why their sex was dwindling, but he could not get a straight answer out of Daniel. Improving their communication skills and reaffirming their faith in a commitment to the relationship helped this couple. Daniel risked expressing his desires to William, and William risked expanding his sexual horizons.

Couples are much easier to treat when the partners are committed and in love. But when they present with significant relational symptoms, one or both partners may not be in love. The couples in which neither partner is in love are short-lived. Consider the following case of Janice and Lee who were constantly fighting.

Janice and Lee met in high school and dated throughout. Although they were inseparable at the time, Lee made it clear to his friends that his intention was to attend college "as far away from his hometown as possible." He found his parents far too intrusive to stay in the area.

Lee admitted that he loved Janice and certainly enjoyed the sex they had together, but he was not interested in extending their relationship beyond high school. His relationship was more out of convenience than romance. Lee said that ever since he told Janice of his intentions, the couple have been fighting nonstop. "She doesn't realize it, but she is making it much easier for me to leave," he said.

Janice had high expectations for the relationship and thought that the couple could prevent separation by attending the same college. She asked Lee to come with her to therapy before he applied to college. During the treatment, it became clear that Lee was not in love and in fact could not wait to move and leave everything behind, including Janice. In the first of two sessions, he admitted that he agreed to come to therapy only to help Janice process their separation. Janice was heartbroken and claimed to be in love with Lee. Nevertheless, Lee left and eventually moved across the country. Janice was referred for further treatment.

### Attachment

Influenced by the work of Bowlby (1958, 1969, 1973, 1980), attachment theorists have found that an infant's experience with their primary caregiver (usually the mother) can help determine the quality of their adult romantic relationships (Ainsworth et al., 1978; Freemen et al., 2023; Hazan & Shaver, 1987). That is, the more secure the mother–infant bond, the better the infant will be able to form adult attachments and make commitments. Longitudinal research has supported this notion (Stanley et al., 2010).

Ainsworth et al. (1978) reported three attachment styles based on an infant's interaction with the primary caregiver: *secure, anxious/ambivalent,* and *avoidant.* Having had a safe and secure attachment to the mother figure – an outgrowth of confidence that the mother figure will be available to meet the infant's needs – the infant has a good chance of growing into a happy, secure adult with the capacity to trust, attach, and commit to others (Ainsworth et al., 1978). In a study conducted by Hazan and Shaver (1987), the relationships of secure individuals were found to last longer (10.02 years compared to 4.86 years for the anxious/ambivalent and 5.97 years for the avoidant individuals). The authors also found that only 6% of secure individuals divorced compared with 10% of anxious/ambivalent and 12% of avoidant individuals.

Infants who experienced inconsistent caregiving or interference in getting one's needs met may develop into an anxious/ambivalent individual. In adult relationships, this type of individual struggles with joining in an intimate relationship and is characterized by both excitement and excruciation. Obsessive jealousy is sometimes present (Ainsworth et al., 1978; Hazan & Shaver, 1987). About commitment in the anxious/ambivalent individual, Freeman et al. (2023) wrote:

> More anxiously attached individuals begin relationships less committed, increase commitment at a slower rate, and peak sooner than their less secure counterparts. In addition, a steeper and sooner descent among more anxious individuals reveals that commitment in the long term has returned to the level of new relationships. In contrast, less insecure individuals in long term relationships report considerably higher commitment levels than their counterparts in new relationships.
>
> (p. 19)

James brought his girlfriend, Kristen, into treatment to convince her to marry him. James thought highly of himself and could not believe Kristen was ambivalent about marrying him. They both admitted that he treated Kristen like a queen and looked after her every need. What was especially puzzling to James was that the couple had passionate sex and that Kristen was extremely jealous of him. Sometimes she would make a scene in public places if she thought another woman was flirting with him or *vice versa*.

After obtaining Kristen's history, I learned that she was abandoned by both her father and her alcoholic mother. She also left a string of men over the years, and many of the relationships were quite volatile. One ex-boyfriend had to get a restraining order to stop her from stalking him. Ironically, however, Kristen routinely dodged her current boyfriend's offer of marriage and was even found to have cheated on him more than once. When her boyfriend first brought Kristen to meet his family, she spent most of the visit vomiting in the bathroom. At the time she claimed to have a virus, but in the treatment, she admitted that she was anxious and later that evening suffered a panic attack, typical of an anxious/ambivalent type.

Having been raised by a cold and distant mother figure, the infant may grow into an avoidant adult who is distrustful and fearful of getting close to others (Ainsworth et al., 1978; Hazan & Shaver, 1987). Neuharth (2018) described these individuals as "commitment shy." The author referred to them as vague, distancing, non-committal, and not fully invested. He also found them to depend on self-reliance rather than interdependence. Robinson et al. (2019) found avoidants to be the opposite of the anxious/ambivalent types. Consider the following example of an avoidant type.

Dan was attracted to his girlfriend, Robin, from the first time he saw her in college. He found her both brilliant and beautiful. After his initial formal introduction to her, he called his mother and told her that he had finally found "the one." But Robin had another prominent characteristic: she was mysterious. She was not keen on expressing herself, and although she thought Dan was a good person to whom she was reasonably attracted, she consistently distanced herself from him, often without warning. Dan described this as "fading." She did this several times during their relationship, and each time Dan had to pursue her and restart the relationship.

Robin saw herself as an independent woman who was raised by her mother to never depend on a man. She planned to have her own career and to live alone if need be. When the couple came for treatment, Robin seemed bothered – as if the process was a waste of her time. She initiated very little conversation and offered vague responses to many of my questions. She seemed to me as if she were in another place, usually her work, which was very important to her and her sense of independence.

### Intimacy

According to the American Psychological Association (2015): "Intimacy characterizes close, familiar and usually affectionate or loving personal relationships and requires the parties to have a detailed knowledge or deep understanding of each other" (p. 558). Schnarch (1991) defined intimacy as "the recursive process of open self-confrontation and disclosure of core aspects of self in the presence of a partner" (p. 121). And Sternberg (1998) referred to intimacy as "feelings of closeness, connectedness, and bondedness in loving relationships" (p. 6).

Intimacy requires partners to be vulnerable with each other. In my clinical experience, partners tend to think that if they can express positive or pleasant information to their mates, they are being intimate. But this is only partially true. The intimate couple can also express negative or critical information freely and without fear of consequences. The following example is that of a couple who had a great deal of difficulty with intimacy.

Jennifer grew up in a home in which "children were to be seen and not heard." She claimed that her parents would be happy to accept compliments from their children, but anything negative was met with outrage. My mother's favorite line in responding to anything she perceived as critical or negative was "After all I've done for you..." Following her marriage to Frank, Jennifer had a great deal of difficulty expressing her point of view, especially if Frank took it as a personal criticism, which he usually did.

Frank grew up in a highly critical environment where all family members constantly ridiculed one another without mercy. This contributed to Frank's sensitivity, and he would lose his temper anytime he was criticized.

This response enabled Jennifer to try and hold her feelings in, until one day she exploded and threatened to divorce Frank unless he went to couples therapy with her.

Mozafari and Xu (2020) claimed that "intimate relationships play an integral role in our lives and influence our emotional well-being, physical health, sense of self, and are important across the life span" (p. 1). Living as Jennifer did, in fear that if she spoke her mind Frank would make her pay, was not healthy emotionally or physically. Jennifer suffered from a host of somatic issues such as stomach distress and excruciating muscle tension. She sometimes had trouble sleeping and instead would roam around the house with a great deal of anxiety. She claimed that for years she was in fear of losing control and from time to time thought of having an affair as a release.

This dynamic was also detrimental to Frank. He lived in fear of being criticized, and his physician told him that his temper was contributing to his high blood pressure. He also experienced a new level of anxiety now that his marriage was in jeopardy.

Frank and Jennifer were proof that the more open and intimate partners are, the less trapped and anxious they feel. They enjoy greater closeness and connection and a healthier lifestyle, and there is less of a reason to commiserate and triangulate (Bowen, 1978) outside individuals.

When couples use the term "intimacy," they usually mean "sex." And while sex is a part of intimacy, the quality of sex between partners is correlated with the level of intimacy and romantic commitment they have in their relationship. The closer and more intimate the couple, the greater the commitment to the relationship and *vice versa*, and the better the couple's sex life (Seiter, 2023).

### Passion

Schnarch (1997) associated *passion* with high desire. Sternberg (1998) wrote: passion is a "state of intense longing for union with the other. Passion is the expression of desires and needs – such as for self-esteem, nurturance, affiliation, dominance, submission, and sexual fulfillment" (p. 9). Passion is usually considered short-term. According to Sternberg, it runs high in the early part of a relationship. While romantic commitment is related to passion, this type of commitment evolves and is considered a long-term process. A committed couple may therefore lack passion, and a passionate couple may lack commitment. The following are examples of each.

Hans and Eva were married for 18 years and had two children. They met in high school and have been together ever since, rarely leaving each other's side except when Hans traveled for work. While the couple presented for treatment to cope with the death of a close relative, during the evaluation it was revealed that the couple had not had sexual relations for 10 years. They did have sex early in the relationship, but because there was never a burning desire to do so on either part, they easily transitioned into what they admitted was a stable, brother–sister relationship. When questioned as to whether this was satisfactory, both said that it was, and that they had a strong desire to keep the family intact; that stability and security were of the utmost importance. They also said that they can be affectionate but what they really value is that they can talk about any subject. If you recall, Hatfield et al. (2008) referred to this type of relationship as "companionate."

Paula and her boyfriend, Kurt, met at a bar and were immediately physically and emotionally attracted. After a four-hour conversation, Paula asked Kurt to sleep with her that night and it was the beginning of a passionate sexual affair. After approximately two years, the couple decided to marry, but despite great sex, they soon found that neither could tolerate being monogamous. Kurt said he felt trapped, and Paula claimed she was bored. The couple sought treatment to discuss opening their marriage, but it soon came out that Paula was already engaged in a sexual relationship with another man and seriously considering ending her relationship with Kurt.

## Further Reflections

### Attachment: The Most Important Ingredient

While the concepts of attachment, love, intimacy, and passion are important ingredients of romantic commitment, not all these ingredients are equally crucial for the survival of a couple. It is nearly impossible to form any kind of romantic commitment without the ability to "attach" to someone. Without attachment, there will be little, if any, intimacy, passion will be short-lived, and love or falling in love will not have a chance to develop. Many couples can and do survive with any one or more of the other ingredients missing. Consider the following cases.

Glenn and his long-term girlfriend, Hallie, had a very intense sex life, full of passion. The couple could not keep their hands off one another, and it all started when they first met in high school. They married as soon as they graduated and have been attached ever since. Both partners said they talk about most things but felt like they could raise their level of intimacy with the help of couples therapy. Hallie specifically complained that sometimes Glenn got too absorbed in his work and neglected her, which Glenn acknowledged. The couple loved one another and were in love. They were also high in emotional and physical attraction and passion. Although they were relatively intimate, they felt they could use some help in that area.

Tony and Sheila, on the other hand, were an older couple who were higher on connection or intimacy but lower on passion. They claimed to love and be in love and to be totally committed to one another. But they wanted to improve their sex life. Tony had experienced some heart problems, which set their sex life back, but now that he was feeling better, the couple need some guidance on how to get back to where they once were. One of the problems was that both partners feared that resuming sex might exacerbate Tony's heart issues. They believed this even though Tony's cardiologist told them they could have sex. Sheila was right when she said that she and Tony had themselves in a rut and did not know how to get out of it.

Even though Glenn and Hallie were low in intimacy and Toby and Sheila were low on passion, neither couple were at risk because they were both high on attachment. Glenn and Hallie have been inseparable since high school, and Toby and Sheila had been together for many years before they experienced symptoms. If either couple had a problem attaching, their symptoms would have been far more serious, or they never would have made it to treatment. Consider the following example of a couple with a severe attachment problem.

Thomas would not admit it, but he was frightened to commit to any woman. In fact, he could not seem to attach to anyone for a prolonged time. His pattern was to go out with a woman until she showed some signs of becoming serious. At this point he would then quickly begin to date someone else, even while sleeping with the first woman. This way he made sure he was committed to neither. Thomas was so adept at his dynamic I asked him why he decided to attend couples therapy with Dale, his latest short-term girlfriend. He coldly said that he was not quite done with Dale but that he was already looking for someone else. True to his word, Thomas began an affair with another women and broke off with Dale in the middle of treatment. As predicted, Thomas could not attach to me either. He moved from therapist to therapist even though we got along well, showing that his inability to attach manifested in many relational contexts.

### Commitment at Risk: When Ingredients Are Missing or Inadequate

Each of the four key ingredients of romantic commitment outlined above must be present in a romantic relationship to some degree or the relationship is vulnerable. This does not mean that the relationship will necessarily end. But when there is a void in a relationship, the relationship is at risk. For example, Don and Sally claimed to love and be in love with each other and to have a great sex life. Don said that he was wildly attracted to Sally the first time he saw her in high school and continues to be. Nevertheless, the couple presented for treatment because they rarely spoke to each other, especially about important or delicate issues. Even when it came to problems with their three children, they usually handled things separately. They could not seem to connect or establish an intimate relationship. Sally mentioned that the couple rarely dated without another couple in tow. And most surprisingly, they even invited three other couples on their honeymoon. Sally admitted she was lonely when she was alone with Don and that she often fantasized about having a partner she could talk to.

Kim claimed that she loved her husband, Richard, but that she was not in love with him. She rarely had sex with him and embarked on a series of affairs. Kim said Richard was a "great guy." She said that she valued him as a friend and confidante and that she was not ready for a divorce. Richard knew his wife was distancing but claimed that her sex drive was never that high and that the kids and her job probably lowered her sex drive. He had no idea this had anything to do with him. Meanwhile Kim withdrew more and more and could no longer even kiss Richard. The couple were high on love and attachment, but low on intimacy and passion, and that made the difference. Kim finally got the nerve to tell Richard she was going to divorce him. He was totally baffled by her decision.

### Commitment and Its Ingredients on a Continuum

Like many other concepts, commitment exists on a continuum from low to high. Couples at the high end of the continuum are more committed and experience fewer symptoms or deficits in key ingredients. Conversely, those couples at the low end of the commitment continuum are less committed and, in turn, reflect the symptoms to support this. Since one partner will appear to be higher on the continuum when they initially present for treatment, the therapist must keep in mind that couples share a conflict with commitment. Even though it may look different at first blush, as discussed in Chapter 2, the truth is that their lack of commitment is relatively equal; it simply manifests differently as one plays the role of the committed and the other plays the role of the uncommitted.

### Development and Commitment

Commitment in a relationship is thought to move through different developmental stages over time. For example, when a young couple begin their relationship, it is usually full of passion and sex is plentiful and spontaneous. You do not hear excuses such as "We no longer have sex because I like it in the evening, and my partner likes it in the morning." Instead, you may hear: "I can't keep my hands off of her," or "I have found my soul mate."

While intimacy usually takes longer to develop, it is common for new partners to report that they speak on the telephone for hours or close many bars or restaurants together.

As the responsibilities of life advance, however, a couple's spontaneity may slowly dissipate and in some instances so does the sex. There seems to be an attempt to exert control over oneself and one's partner. It is now more likely to hear something like: "We can't have sex when the kids are in the house. I just cannot relax," or "He doesn't kiss me anymore the way he used to."

If a couple can replace this lack of spontaneity with greater connection and grow their intimacy, they can survive. But it is not unusual for intimacy to dissipate as well. I was sitting in a restaurant, and I noticed that a middle-aged, married couple at the table next to me did not say a word to each other for the entire meal. They each told the waitress what they wanted to eat and then proceeded to stare at their cell phones until they had finished their meals. The only words uttered between them were spoken at the very end of the meal when the husband asked his wife: "Are you ready to go?"

Many couples are held together by obligations, and love supplants the feeling of being in love. As a result of these changes, the strength of their once unquestionable commitment may fray, and symptoms begin to show in key areas such as passion and intimacy. How high a couple is on the commitment continuum when they first join together helps to determine how the couple will fare over time. If, for example, a couple have a very strong commitment when they first come together, the longer the passion and intimacy that they initially felt will last.

## References

Ackerman, J. M., Griskevicius, V., & Li, N. P. (2011). Let's get serious: Communicating commitment in romantic relationships. *Journal of Personality and Social Psychology, 100*, 1079–1094. https://doi.org/10.1037/a0022412

Agnew, C. (2009). Commitment: Theories and typologies. *Department of Psychological Sciences Faculty Publications*. Paper 28. https://docs.lib.purdue.edu/psychpubs/28/

Ainsworth, M. D. S., Blehar, M. C., Waters, E., & Wall, S. N. (1978). *Patterns of attachment: A psychological study of the strange situation*. Erlbaum.

Aman, J., Abbas, J., Nurunnabi, M., & Bano, S. (2019). The relationship of religiosity and marital satisfaction: The role of religious commitment and practices on marital satisfaction among Pakistani respondents. *Sustainability, 9*, 1–23. https://dx.doi.org/10.3390/su11061683.marriages

Amato, R. R., & Hohmann-Marriott, B. (2007). A comparison of high- and low-distress marriages that end in divorce. *Journal of Marriage and Family Therapy, 69*, 621–638.

American Psychological Association (2015). *APA dictionary of psychology* (2nd ed.). APA.

Bieber, C., & Ramirez, A. (2024, January). Revealing divorce statistics in 2024. *Forbes Advisor*. https://www.forbes.com/advisor/leal/divorce/divorce-statistics/

Bowen, M. (1978). *Family therapy in clinical practice*. Aronson.

Bowlby, J. (1958). The nature of the child's tie to his mother. *International Journal of Psychanalysis, 39*, 350–373.

Bowlby, J. (1969). *Attachment and loss: Vol. 1. Attachment* (2nd ed.). Basic Books.

Bowlby, J. (1973). *Attachment and loss: Vol. 2. Separation: Anxiety and anger* (2nd ed.). Basic Books.

Bowlby, J. (1980). *Attachment and loss: Vol. 3. Loss: Sadness and depression* (2nd ed.). Basic Books.

Buss, D. (2019). The evolution of love in humans. In R. J. Sternberg & K. Sternberg (Eds.), *The new psychology of love* (pp. 42–63). Cambridge University Press.

Cervini, R. (2023, June). Unveiling the four types of commitment: Building stronger bonds. Retrieved from https://ricardocervini.medium.com/unveiling-the-four-types-of-commitment-building-stronger-bonds--ec4c1e305

Clark, H. H. (2006). Social actions, social commitments. In S. Levinson & N. J. Enfield (Eds.), *Roots of human sexuality* (pp. 126–150). Routledge.

Day, M. V., Kay, A. C., Holmes, J. G., & Napier, J. L. (2011). System justification and the defense of committed relationship ideology. *Journal of Personality and Social Psychology, 101*, 291–306. https://doi.org/10.1037/a0023197

Fehr, B. (2012). Stability and commitment in friendships. In J. M. Adams & W. H. Jones (Eds.), *Handbook of interpersonal commitment and relationship stability* (pp. 259–280). Spring Science + Business Media, LLC.

Fisher, H. (2004). *Why we love: The nature and chemistry of romantic love*. Henry Holt.

Freeman, H., Simons, J., & Benson, N. F. (2023). Romantic duration, relationship quality, and attachment insecurity among dating couples. *International Journal of Environmental Research and Public Health, 20*, 1–18. https://doi.org/10.3390/ijerph20010856

Gillette, H. (2022). The top 12 reasons for divorce. *PsychCentral*. https://psychcentral.com/relationships/top-reasons-for-divorce

Gillis, K. (2023, August). Love vs in love – The difference between love and in love according to a therapist. https://www.choosingtherapy.com/love-vs-in-love

Gold Buscho, A. (2021, May). The 3 most common preventable reasons people divorce: Most causes of divorce are preventable. Here are the solutions. Psychology Today. https://www.psychologytoday.com/intl/blog/better-divorce/202105/the-3-most-common-preventable-reasons-people-divorce

Gómez-López, M., Viejo, C., & Ortega-Ruiz, R. (2019). Well-being and romantic relationships: A systemic review in adolescence and emerging adulthood. *International Journal of Environmental Research and Public Health, 16*, 1–31. https://doi.org/10.3390/ijerph16132415

Gregor-Planer, D. (2019). The relationship between organizational commitment and organizational citizenship behaviors in the public and private sectors. *Sustainability, 11*, 2–20. https://doi.org/10.3390/su11226395

Harrison, M. A. (2022). Emotional commitment. In T. K. Shackelford (Ed.), *The Cambridge handbook of evolutionary perspectives on sexual psychology* (Vol. 3, pp. 399–425). Cambridge University Press.

Hatfield, E. C., Pillemer, J. T., O'Brien, M. U., & Le, Y.-C. L. (2008). The endurance of love: Passionate and companionate love in newlywed and long-term marriages. *Interpersona: An International Journal on Personal Relationships, 2*, 35–64. https://doi.org/10.5964/ijpr.v2i1.17

Hatfield, E. C., & Walster, G. W. (1978). *A new look at love; a revealing report on the most elusive of all emotions.* University Press of America.

Hazan, C., & Shaver, P. (1987). Romantic love conceptualized as an attachment process. *Journal of Personality and Social Psychology, 52*, 511–524. https://doi.org/10.1037/0022-3514.52.3.511

Johnson, M. P. (2012). Personal, moral, and structural commitment to relationships: Experiences of choice and constraint. In J. M. Adams & W. H. Jones (Eds.), *Handbook of interpersonal commitment and relationship stability* (pp. 73–87). Spring Science + Business Media, LLC.

Jones, M. A. (2018). Strong social networks are key to turning around communities. *Stanford Social Innovation Review.* Retrieved from https://ssir.org/articles/entry/strong_social_networks_are_key_to_turning_around_communities

Kochar, R. K., & Sharma, D. (2015). Role of love in relationship satisfaction. *The International Journal of Indian Psychology, 3*, 81–107. https://doi.org/10.25215/0301.102

Lindner, J. (2024, June). Must-know reasons for divorce statistics. *Gitnux Market Data Report* 2024. https://gitnux.org/reasons-for-divorce-statistics

Londero-Santos, A., Natividade, J. C., & Féres-Carniero, T. (2021). Do romantic relationships promote happiness: Relationships' characteristics as predictors of subjective well-being. *Journal of Personal Relationships, 15*, 3–19. https://doi.org/10.5964/ijpr.4195

Lovering, N. (2022). The psychology of love. *PsychCentral.* Retrieved from https://psychcentral.com/relationships/the-psychology-of-love

McCoy, K. (2018, June). In love versus loving. *Psychology Today.* https://www.psychologytoday.com/us/blog/complicated-love/201806/in-love-versus-loving

Meyer, J. P., Stanley, D. J., Herscovitch, L., & Topolnytsky, L. (2002). Affective continuance, and normative commitment to the organization: A meta-analysis of antecedents, correlates, and consequences. *Journal of Vocational Behavior, 6*, 20–52. https://doi.org/10.1006/jvbe.2001.1842

Michael, J., Sebanz, N., & Knoblich, G. (2015). The sense of commitment: A minimal approach. Frontiers in Psychology, 6. https://doi.org/10.3389/fpsyg.2015.01968

Morgan, H. J., & Shaver, P. R. (2012). Attachment processes and commitment to romantic relationships. In J. M. Adams & W. H. Jones (Eds.), *Handbook of interpersonal commitment and relationship stability* (pp. 109–124). Spring Science + Business Media, LLC.

Mozafari, P. R., & Xu, X. (2020). Intimate relationships. In F. M. Cheung & D. F. Halpern (Eds.), *The Cambridge handbook of the international psychology of women* (pp. 342–354). Cambridge University Press.

Neuharth, D. (2018, July). 16 signs of an avoidant or unavailable partner. *PsychCentral*. https://psychcentral.com/blog/love—matters/2018/07/16-signs-of-an-avoidant-or-unavailable-partner1

Rill, L., Baiocchi-Wagner, E. A., Denker, K., & Olson, L. N. (2009). Exploration of the relationship between self-esteem, commitment, and verbal aggressiveness in romantic dating relationships. Communication Reports, *22*, 102–113. https://doi.org/10.1080/0893421090361587

Robinson, L., Segal, J., & Jaffe, J. (2019). Attachment styles and how they affect adult relationships. *Helpguide.org*. https://www.helpguide.org/relationships/social-connection/attachment-and-adult-relationships

Rusbult, C. E. (1983). A longitudinal test of the investment model: The development (and deterioration) of satisfaction and commitment in heterosexual involvements. *Journal of Personality and Social Psychology, 45*, 101–117. https://doi.org/10.1037/0022-3514.45.1.101

Rusbult, C. E., & Farrell, D. (1983). A longitudinal test of the investment model: The impact on job satisfaction, job commitment, and turnover of variations in rewards, costs, alternatives, and investments. *Journal of Applied Psychology, 68*, 429–438. https://doi.org/10.1037/0021-9010.68.3.429

Schnarch, D. (1991). *Constructing the sexual crucible: An integration of sexual and marital therapy*. Norton.

Schnarch, D. (1997). *Passionate marriage: Sex, love. and intimacy in emotionally committed relationships*. Norton.

Schoebi, D., Karney, B. R., & Bradbury, T. N. (2012). Stability and change in the first 10 years of marriage. Does commitment confer benefits beyond the effects of satisfaction? *Journal of Personality and Social Psychology, 102*, 729–742.

Scott, S. B., Rhoades, G. K., Stanley, S. M., Allen, E. S., & Markman, H. J. (2013). Reasons for divorce and recollections of premarital interventions: Implications for improving relationship education. *Couple and Family Psychology, 2*, 131–145. https://doi.org/10.1037/90032025

Seiter, T. (2023, July). How to get more commitment and better your sex life: Want commitment? Work on your sex life. Want a better sex life? Get committed. *Psychology Today*. https://www.psychologytoday.com/us/blog/mindful-relationships/202307/how-to-get-more-commitment-and-better-your-sex-life

Stanley, S. M., & Markman, H. J. (1992). Assessing commitment in personal relationships. *Journal of Marriage and Family, 54*, 595–608. https://doi.org/10.2307/353245

Stanley, S. M., Rhoades, G. K., & Whitton, S. W. (2010). Commitment: Functions, formation, and securing of romantic attachment. *Journal of Family Therapy Review, 2*, 243–257. https://doi.org/10.1111/J.1756.2010.00060.x

Sternberg, R. J. (1998). *Cupid's arrow: The course of love through time*. Cambridge.

Sternberg, R. J. (2019). When love goes awry (Part 1): Applications of the duplex theory of love and its development to relationships gone bad. In R. J. Sternberg & K. Sternberg (Eds.), *The new psychology of love* (2nd ed., pp. 280–299). Cambridge University Press.

Surra, C. A., Hughes, D. K., & Jacquet, S. E. (2012). The development of commitment to marriage: A phenomenological approach. In J. M. Adams & W. H.

Jones (Eds.), *Handbook of interpersonal commitment and relationship stability* (pp. 125–148). Spring Science + Business Media, LLC.

Thomas, P. A., Lui, H., & Umberson, D. (2017). Family relationships and well-being. *Innovation in Aging, 1,* 1–11. https://doi.org/10.1093/geroni/igx025

Van der Heijden, B. I. J. M., Davies, E. M. M., Van der Linden, D., Bozionelos, N., & De Vos, A. (2022). The relationship between career commitment and career success among university staff: The mediating role of employability. *European Management Review, 19,* 564–580. https://doi.org/10.1111/emre.12503

Weir, K. (2018). Life-saving relationships. *Monitor on Psychology, 49,* 46. American Psychological Association.

Wiecha, J. (2023). Emotional commitment: Relationship satisfaction. In T. K. Shackelford (Ed.), *Encyclopedia of sexual psychology and behavior* (pp. 1–6). Springer.

Wilson, E. O. (2000). *Sociobiology: The new synthesis, twenty-fifth anniversary edition.* Belknap Press of Harvard University Press.

# Chapter 2

# Romantic Commitment

## Types and Tendencies

Often a couple will present for treatment with at least one partner "demonstrating" less of a commitment to the relationship than the other (Stanley, 2016). That is, the partner who claims to want commitment relentlessly pursues the other for it usually in the contexts of love, attachment, intimacy, or passion. The other partner may be slow to respond, prone to distance, or neglectful and abusive – anything to back the committed partner off. This begs the question: If one truly desires commitment, why then engage with someone who does not or is incapable of it? Is the seemingly committed partner also commitment-avoidant, by pairing with someone who cannot commit?

Usually, the partner who appears to be committed is unaware of their low commitment and attributes the couple's symptoms to their partner. The noncommitted partner, however, may be conscious or at least somewhat aware that they are not very committed to the relationship. Whether they realize it or not, their mutual low commitment is likely responsible for their relationship symptoms, which may manifest in insufficient love, attachment, intimacy, and passion. Consider the following list and note that while the committed–uncommitted dynamic appears complementary, so too are the pairings that represent these differences (see Figure 2.1). I have only listed the types and tendencies I have seen most often in my clinical practice. Some may overlap, but they are different enough to mention. I will first address the committed partner.

## The Committed

### The Pursuer

Some who are unconditionally committed to their relationships worry so much about losing their indifferent partners that they pursue them at every turn. They might constantly check their cell phones or computers to see where they are or who they are talking to. Many follow them and some

DOI: 10.4324/9781003475743-3

| Presents Committed | Presents Uncommitted |
|---|---|
| Pursuer | Distancer |
| Anxious/Dependent | Disengaged |
| Selfless, Pleaser | Selfish, Narcissist |
| Loyal, Trustworthy | Disloyal, Untrustworthy |
| Low Self-esteem | Pseudo Confident |
| Masochist | Sadist |
| Transactional | Transactional |

*Figure 2.1* Committed – Uncommitted Complementary Pairs.

hire private detectives. These individuals want to be attached to their partners and feel quite anxious when they are not by their sides. This smothering effect often chases the noncommitted partner even further away and is reminiscent of the oft-written-about pursuer–distancer dynamic (Betchen, 2004; Fogarty, 1979).

Stan had been married to Lindsay for several years, but he acted completely indifferent toward her in all contexts of their relationship. He tried to avoid being alone with her, and when he was with her, he ignored her. Rather than take the hint, Lindsay chose to relentlessly pursue Stan but to no avail. In fact, the only thing that kept Stan in the same house was Lindsay's decision to give him lots of sex. Stan admitted that he got more sex than any of his friends, but he felt no attraction or passion toward Lindsay. He described sex as a mechanical exercise that served as a release.

Stan and Lindsay were void of intimacy, and the more Lindsay pursued, the less Stan paid her any attention. Lindsay desperately wanted Stan but knew he did not want her. She, however, could not give up trying to win him over. She called him several times a day at work and was constantly trying to arrange dates for the two of them.

### The Anxious/Dependent

People with a low tolerance for being alone are likely to take whatever comes along out of a sense of anxious desperation. Unfortunately, because they are so desperate, they are likely to be taken advantage of or to tolerate far more abuse or neglect than they should in their relationships. Ironically, this type of individual seeks security and is dependent but chooses someone less likely to commit to them.

Iris admittedly was an anxious woman. She grew up with two alcoholic parents and little financial security. She suffered from panic attacks from time to time and was in constant fear that her husband, Ray, would leave her. Although Ray often acted indifferent to Iris and her needs – he even laughed at her when she caught him in an affair with a work colleague – Iris would rationalize and say that Ray might not be a great husband, but given what she had experienced in life, he is still the best thing that's ever happened to her. Iris was caught between her need for stability and security and her uncommitted husband.

### The Selfless, Pleaser

Selfless people tend to ignore their own needs and focus on the needs of others. When they are mistreated or ignored, the first person they tend to question or blame is themselves. This style allows them to choose a partner who is indifferent toward them. Again, they dislike being taken advantage of but are far too much of a pleaser to set limits or escape their situation. I have found that many of these individuals have a strong need to be loved and desired and will go to great lengths to win a partner's approval even though this has been proven to be a futile act.

Helen was a beautiful woman, and her new husband, Ed, could not believe his good fortune in marrying her. However, Helen knew that she was beautiful and that most men wanted her. She also thought that she could have chosen a better-looking and richer man but instead she settled for Ed. She felt that she was getting old and should finally commit to somebody. Helen was not interested in having sex with Ed, and she continued to flirt with other men as if she were single. She believed that she was so valued by Ed that he would not dare demand that she curbs her solicitous behavior. Instead of setting limits with Helen, however, Ed relentlessly tried to find more ways to please her, none of which worked. Ed admitted he had always been a selfless pleaser and that Helen could get him to do anything.

### The Loyal, Trustworthy

Some people are loyal and trusting to a fault. This type of individual may find it hard to believe, for example, that their partner is misbehaving or betraying them despite evidence to the contrary. They can also become enraged with anyone who tries to tell them the truth and might cut them out of their lives indefinitely. Unfortunately, when reality penetrates this individual's defenses, they may become traumatized. It is as if their world has been turned upside down and they are losing all control.

Ginny knew that her fiancé, Todd, had a history of cheating on every woman he had been with, including two women he was previously engaged to. She heard this directly from some of these women who were only too glad to help Ginny from becoming "Todd's next victim," as one put it. But Ginny saw Todd as totally committed and trustworthy. Even when her sister caught Todd with another woman, she didn't accept her sister's findings. Instead, she accused her sister of being jealous and trying to sabotage her impending marriage to Todd. On her wedding day, Ginny mistakenly walked in on Todd having sex with one of her bridesmaids. Ginny was so distraught she fainted and soon had to be medicated and hospitalized. Even with treatment, however, it took some time for Ginny to stop questioning whether she saw correctly that day.

### Those with Low Self-Esteem/Low Self-Worth

People who feel inferior or think little of themselves are more likely to expose themselves to situations in which they will be taken advantage of. These individuals might not be masochistic, but they tend to believe that they are not good enough for their partners. Whatever morsel the uncommitted partner offers is welcomed. This type of individual claims to want to be treated better but does not feel deserving of such treatment.

Before they even dated, Keith told Karen that he knew she did not like him that much, but if she gave him a chance, he would do anything for her. He even told her he would allow her to date other men if she dated him. Karen took Keith up on his offer and dated him for two years, cheating on him regularly, until she broke up with him. Keith, however, said he did not regret his decision to date Karen. He knew the day would come when she would leave him, but he still thought the deal he made with her was worth the limited time spent with her and the humiliation it brought.

Pete was a laborer with a high school education who worked as a maintenance man in a factory. When he attended treatment, he brought with him his young, vivacious wife who held two masters' degrees and worked as a management consultant in a large corporation. The differences between their ages and level of energy were obvious as were their educational and intellectual levels.

Pete told me in an individual session that he knew Karen would one day leave him, but if he lasted five years in the relationship, he would be satisfied. He said Karen made him a better person and improved his life far more than he could imagine. He said that he felt as if she was his superior. He claimed that he was in love with Karen but that living with her was very stressful. He said that she had high expectations and he constantly felt pressure to improve himself. He wanted to tell her this, but he feared that if he challenged her authority and superiority, she might leave him sooner.

### The Masochist

There are some individuals who, no matter how poorly they are treated, demonstrate an incredibly high tolerance and a misplaced sense of loyalty to their partner and the relationship. In my experience these individuals cope by dissociating or holding on to the fantasy that things will improve. In my experience, some of these individuals qualify as masochists in the nonsexual sense of the term.

Masochists may complain about how they are treated but seem to be attracted to the abuse. According to the American Psychological Association (2015), they "obtain gratification or freedom from guilt feelings as a consequence of humiliation, self-derogation, self-sacrifice, wallowing in misery, and, in some instances, submitting to physically sadistic act" (p. 625). In this context abuse represents a lack of commitment to the relationship. Consider the following example.

Ken was openly having an affair with a local woman, and he made it clear that he did not care how his wife, Nancy, felt about it. Nancy, however, was extremely upset and desperate. She vacillated between crying, begging, and demanding that Ken end the affair, but he wouldn't. Ken, in fact, simpered when Nancy expressed pain.

Nancy also began to suffer migraines, and her colitis was flaring up. But Ken showed no empathy or remorse. He made it clear that he was considering ending the marriage, but the timing was not quite right. When Nancy was questioned about ending her marriage, she answered that no one in her family ever divorced and that she was not going to be the first even if it killed her. It looked like it might just do that.

Kelly and Tim had been married for several years and had two special needs children who were a great strain on them and their marriage. To make matters worse, Tim was little help and began to drink heavily. Kelly said that she was already ashamed because she did not give birth to two healthy children, but if divorced with two special needs kids, her family and friends would think of her as a "horrible, selfish person." Kelly suffered from severe migraines, and none of her medical treatments seemed to work. But she could not risk the stigma attached to extricating herself from her situation.

### The Transactional

Transactional relationships are like business deals. They also tend to be short on emotion, passion, and intimacy; the sex may even be purpose driven and robotic. Two highly ambitious people may mate for the primary purpose of helping one another achieve. When this plot fails, however, the marriage may be in serious jeopardy. Or consider the wealthy man who chooses a "trophy" wife to impress his friends and to build his ego. He may do this at the expense of having little in common with her.

One good example of a transactional relationship is the "arranged marriage." Couples who come from countries that support arranged marriages have a certain loyalty to their heritage and therefore have a harder time extracting themselves from an untenable situation. They worry not only about what their parents think but their communities as well. If these couples remain in their countries of origin, the culture may bind them no matter the quality of their relationship. If, however, they move to a more open country, they become more vulnerable. Many of these unions are less like relationships and more like business deals.

Raj and Preeti were arranged to be married in India by their families. Although Raj was excited about the match, Preeti was somewhat skeptical. She did not like the concept of arranged marriage and its associated values and norms. She was also not as attracted to Raj and did not think he was very intelligent. But Preeti did not want to disappoint her parents and her community, so she agreed to the match and demonstrated her dissatisfaction by complaining about Raj at every turn. Apparently, he was never able to satisfy her. Raj, however, was very attracted to Preeti and did not think that he could ever find anyone as smart and pretty like her. He wanted to marry her the first time he saw her. Raj knew that Preeti was not as taken with him as he was of her, but he said that he was willing to put up with her behavior – some of which was cruel – to please his parents and maintain cultural traditions. Raj said that a divorce would be humiliating, especially for his parents. He said he was committed to Preeti for life.

Edward was a wealthy but depressed divorcee in his 60s. After a period of unsuccessful dating – which he blamed on the modern American woman's need to be dominant – he was recommended by a friend to look overseas where he said women were subservient to men. Taking his friend's advice, Edward chose what he thought was his perfect match from a mail-order catalog: Natasha, a beautiful, poor, Russian woman 20 years his junior, who was desperate for a husband and a better life.

Agreeing to meet, Edward flew Natasha to the United States, and the couple instantly moved in together and soon married. While the first years of the relationship went well – with Edward showering Natasha with whatever her heart desired – after approximately five years, she wanted out. In fact, she told Edward this the day after her college graduation. By then Natasha had obtained her citizenship, an education paid for by Edward, and a good job.

Edward was stunned and even more depressed than he was before he met Natasha. He could not believe that she was willing to give up the luxurious life he had provided for her. He claimed to have been committed to Natasha for the rest of his life. Nevertheless, Natasha filed for divorce and got a sizeable settlement from her wealthy American husband. Apparently, Edward failed to insist on a pre-nuptial agreement.

## The Uncommitted

### The Distancer

Some people avoid closeness. Whether it is to avert a potentially volatile confrontation, or the discomfort of commitment to one's partner, these individuals would rather run away than deal with their issues directly. Distancers can emotionally or physically distance. In a romantic relationship, for example, they may fail to initiate sex, remember birthdays, or complement their partners – basically anything that might encourage closeness and full commitment. They want to be in relationships but require a certain amount of space between them and their partners. Consider the following example of a classic distancer.

Kirk was a good example of a distancer I can remember. Although he had been married to his wife, Jessica, for over 18 years, he never once told her she was beautiful or that he loved her. He also routinely forgot to celebrate significant holidays such as her birthday or Valentine's Day.

Jessica pursued Kirk, mostly by complaining, but recently she was threatening to end the marriage if he didn't spend more time with her. Kirk said that he understood Jessica's complaint about him and that he wanted to be with her, but he said that she was too much. He said that she wanted to talk all the time and insisted he go deeper into certain subjects. He said that what Jessica was asking of him felt uncomfortable. He added that he needed to regulate the closeness between them so that they didn't get "swallowed up by it."

### The Disengaged

The disengaged type is closely related to the distancer but different enough to mention. Whereas the distancer moves away from a partner, they may still care or have compassion for them. Distancers can still love and be in love, and there can be times of passion and intimacy. They simply cannot tolerate too much closeness and have a need to put space between themselves and their partners. I view the disengaged as an individual who is checked out emotionally and physically, full-time.

Sal claimed that his wife, Samantha, of 12 years, was never present. He described her as "a million miles away." Even when the couple have sex, which is not frequent, Sal complained that it was robotic and passionless. He also reported that Samantha rarely engages him in conversation. He not only has to initiate talks with her, but she rarely responds with more than a short answer. Sal said that when Samantha looks at him, it is as if she is "staring right through me."

### The Selfish, Narcissist

Some people form relationships or marry to primarily have their needs met. A selfless mate, which is who they seek out, will cater to them and help build their ego. A wealthy, selfless partner can meet their materialistic needs as well. Selfish, narcissistic people appear to think highly of themselves and can be very critical of others to make themselves feel superior. These individuals are simply too busy trying to improve their lot than worry about such things as love or being in love with a partner. They tend to view relationships as stepping-stones for their own purposes rather than a durable commitment.

Andrea said that she would attend one session with John, but that she had made up her mind to leave him. Heartbroken, John desperately tried to convince her to stay, even promising that she did not have to have sex with him. The couple reported that their relationship had always suffered from a lack of passion and intimacy. But for the last couple of years, Andrea had significantly increased her distancing behavior.

John was from a wealthy family, and Andrea's family struggled financially. John's friends and parents told him repeatedly that Andrea never loved him and that as soon as she could get away with a sizeable divorce settlement, she would leave. There was some truth in this because Andrea could not identify a reason for leaving John other than she was bored.

John suspected Andrea of having an affair with a wealthy man whom she worked with, which Andrea denied. She made it a point to say that she wasn't after John's money and that she wanted a fair and amicable divorce. But John claimed that she had hired one of the most expensive divorce attorneys in the area and was seeking sizeable alimony and more than half of their substantial assets.

### The Disloyal, Untrustworthy

Some people cannot be trusted. Their loyalty is to themselves first and foremost. Some of these individuals are so stealth that their partners have no idea what they are plotting. Usually, they have a history of betrayal, deceit, lies, and secrets. They tend to prey on the naive.

Another feature of this type is that they tend to project their distrust onto others and thus have a difficult time risking commitment. These individuals range from the cautious to the paranoid. Because of their great distrust, they tend to expect the worst from their potential partners and might fear if they commit, they will be taken advantage of. These people may end a relationship before they can be disappointed or hurt.

Fran was slow to trust anyone. She had a series of short-lived relationships with men who labeled her "crazy and paranoid." Apparently, however, it was revealed in treatment that Fran was hypervigilant for fear of being taken advantage of, which then manifested in a need to play detective in her relationships. However, it was not just significant transgressions that Fran was looking out for. Even something minor was perceived as a sign that something bigger and more dangerous lies ahead.

When Fran finally got the nerve to marry, for example, she would look through her husband Evan's wallet, cell phone, and computer. If he purchased a pair of sneakers without telling her, she would accuse him of being a liar, capable of cheating. She would then punish him by not speaking to him, withdrawing sex, and threatening to end the relationship. The more she distrusted, however, the less forthright Evan was with her.

### The Pseudo Confident

The partner who presents as uncommitted will appear more confident than the committed one, who may doubt his or her self-worth. Looking and acting the part for the pseudo confident can serve as a defense against feeling weak. A colleague of mine believes that the indifferent partner in a relationship holds the power. No doubt, the less invested are more in control, but some uncommitted partners cover up low self-esteem, which they hope to remedy through their mate. Perhaps their mate has a more prestigious job or is far more physically attractive. Unfortunately, this reason for entering a serious relationship with someone is not a basis for a durable commitment. This is because as soon as the uncommitted partner achieves any sense of real confidence, they may look for a more suitable partner – one they can experience love and passion with.

Mary was raised in a lower-middle-class family. Her father was a janitor at the local high school, and her mother was a school cook. But despite her humble background, Mary acted as if she came from royalty. She was opinionated and hyperconfident. Despite not having a college education, Mary was quick to debate someone with an advanced degree who specialized in the area and never let her background handicap her. In fact, Mary used her background to fuel her confidence and ambition.

Mary was also blessed with extremely good looks, and some men and women were intimidated by her. When her husband, Gary, a quiet, self-contained man first saw Mary, he instantly fell for her. He was attracted to her physical appearance, confidence, and energy; he liked an out-spoken woman. Mary also happened to be far more advanced sexually than Gary and found him easy to seduce – something Gary did not mind until Mary's sexual passion began to wane.

In comparison to Mary's family, Gary was from great wealth. His parents had a strong sense of tradition and did not think that Mary and their son were an appropriate match. Gary was intimidated by his parents who had a lot of control over him.

While Mary did seem to enjoy her newfound status, she eventually began to view Gary and his friends as critical, snobbish elitists. And while Gary did his best to include Mary in all family activities, she continued to pull away from the relationship, eventually having an affair with a physician.

Gary could not believe that Mary betrayed him. He thought that he had given her everything that she had always fantasized about in life. Soon, however, he realized Mary was just using him to elevate her stature and raise her self-esteem; she was never committed to their marriage. During their separation process, Mary even admitted to not liking Gary and his family, but she did appreciate him introducing her to "how the other half lives."

### The Sadist

Those who were never interested in commitment and feel trapped in one may become mean and abusive. They may name call, flirt with others in front of their partners, humiliate partners in public, or even physically discipline them. Some of these individuals may qualify as sadistic or those who obtain some form of "pleasure through cruelty" (American Psychological Association, 2015, p. 930). Consider the case of Jane.

Jane, recently out of a dysfunctional, long-term relationship, was struggling to find a path forward. Even with two graduate degrees, she was unclear about her future. When she first met Kevin, she felt no emotional or physical attraction toward him but thought he would vastly improve her dire life. Kevin also happened to be needy. He had gone through a taxing divorce and was admittingly lonely and anxious to start over.

The couple married after approximately three months of dating, but Kevin's affluence could not make up for Jane's lack of attraction. The relationship was therefore void of intimacy and passion, and within a year, Jane began lashing out at Kevin every chance she got. Kevin tried to please Jane, but no effort was sufficient. Jane berated and emasculated him both at home and in public and frequently referred to him as a "loser." Kevin could not even make their bed to her liking.

### The Transactional

A transaction usually entails an expectation of mutual reciprocity or a *quid pro quo*. A transactional romantic relationship is less about love and intimacy and more about the "deal." I'm sure you have heard the saying: "It's nothing personal, it's just business." Most often an uncommitted partner will enter a relationship primarily to survive or to thrive, not because of attraction, love, or to achieve intimacy. Whether this partner is aware of it or not, he or she has no intention of commitment. After getting what they want, they may leave the relationship.

Sophia married Matthew soon after they met, but she admitted in an individual session that she was never in love with him. She saw him as a vehicle to obtain a college education so that she could secure a job and a life of her own apart from him. The relationship interaction resembled a business deal or transaction. The couple were cordial to each other, but there was very little affection, especially on Sophia's part. In fact, when Matthew would touch her arm or thigh during a session, she would quickly pull his hand away.

The couple had sporadic sex, but Sophia treated it like an occasional obligation or payment for services rendered. Matthew confirmed that during the act she appeared disinterested with a desire to get it over with. He claimed there was little love or passion from her end. The couple rarely conversed and admitted they had little interpersonal connection.

Despite this couple's dynamic, Matthew took care of all Sophia's needs, especially financially. He was not happy with his relationship, and he wanted more from Sophia, but he felt that the little she gave was better than nothing.

People may form long-term relationships or marry because they think they will then be perceived as normal and may also be in a transactional relationship. This is one reason gay people marry straight people. But this dynamic is fraught with internal and external conflict. In my clinical experience, when an individual is not in a relationship where they can be true to themselves, there may be basic love but rarely is there intimacy, passion, a feeling of being in love, and durable commitment.

Joseph and Allison were a married couple with two young children. They came for treatment because Joseph had been distancing for quite some time. Once a great father, according to Allison, he rarely spent time with their kids, and on more than one occasion, he did not come home after work.

After a couple of sessions, Joseph admitted that he had met someone but had yet to consummate the relationship. He said that he loved his wife and children but could no longer live with them. Allison was distraught and asked Joseph if she knew the woman. In response, Joseph shocked her once again by revealing that it was a man he knew from high school. Allison then asked Joseph when he first realized that he was gay. Joseph said that he considered the possibility in high school but was too desperate to fit in. He said that for years he had a homophobic response to gays to ward off his true self.

## References

American Psychological Association (2015). *APA dictionary of psychology* (2nd ed.). APA.

Betchen, S. (2004). *Intrusive partners elusive mates: The pursuer-distancer dynamic in couples*. Routledge.

Fogarty, T. (1979). The distancer and the pursuer. *The Family, 11*, 7–16.

Stanley, S. M. (2016, November). What happens when partners aren't equally committed: New study examines relationships where one is just not into the other. *Psychology Today*. https://www.psychologytoday.com/us/blog/sliding-vs-deciding/201611/what-happens-when-partners-arent-equally-committed

# Chapter 3

# Romantic Commitment and Conflict

## Internal Conflict

When most people hear the word *conflict* in the context of a relationship, they usually think of a disagreement between partners or an *external conflict*. Of most concern here, however, is *internal conflict* or a conflict that exists within an individual – a psychological duality or split between what an individual desires and what they feel comfortable achieving. Some individuals may be aware of both sides of their conflict, but most are only conscious of one side – usually the side that fits with their defenses. They are usually unaware of the other counterintuitive side.

Fred admitted that he wanted to be successful in his career, but he could not admit that there was a side of him that was uncomfortable with success. For example, I once suggested that he may have sabotaged his chances of getting a promotion at work. But he saw this as nonsensical and adamantly refused to accept responsibility. "That does not make any sense," he said. "Why would I want to sabotage my career when I want to be successful so badly?" It was as if he was dissociating from the side of the conflict that preferred failure.

If challenged enough, Fred would revert to blaming his boss or company policy for his failures. It is this counterintuitive side of the conflict that presents the more effective defense against fully comprehending the power and influence of an internal conflict; it is therefore the side that clients unconsciously protect regardless of the consequences.

Even the healthiest of people have conflicts, and when both sides are reasonably balanced, the conflict produces few if any symptoms. That is, when an individual can maintain a psychological equilibrium so that neither side of the conflict dominates the other for too long, the conflict is balanced. If Fred allowed one of his relationships to succeed or he got too close to success, the need for success in this context would dominate. If he constantly failed, however, as he often did, the need to sabotage would

DOI: 10.4324/9781003475743-4

dominate. This notion made sense because Fred would experience anxiety and depression either way.

This way of thinking often baffles clients and therapists alike. But when a conflict dramatically shifts, it usually causes a dramatic reaction. This same dynamic can cause difficulty in a couple when one partner loses a significant amount of weight or a partner becomes famous. The system that kept whatever conflict they had in balance is suddenly thrown off.

Another idiosyncrasy of internal conflict is that even when something positive happens, it may have its consequences. Perhaps this is no more evident than with some lottery winners. Lottery winners with an internal conflict about winning might suffer symptoms if their conflict is unbalanced by a big win. For example, lottery winners would not have played the lottery to begin with if they did not have a desire to improve their lives. But they are uncomfortable with suddenly becoming rich. It is as if buying the lottery ticket represents one side of the conflict ("I'd like to be rich") and winning represents the other side ("I'm uncomfortable being rich"). The fantasy of winning feels better and is less complicated than the reality of winning. While some studies have found that winning the lottery can have a long-term positive impact on life satisfaction (Lindqvist et al., 2020), others have found that it can bring on anxiety, emotional struggles, guilt, a loss of motivation, and a loss of purpose (Bennett, 2023). I suspect the latter were more likely to have been in conflict; some might even give their money away to re-balance their conflict.

Conflicts are deeply lodged in our unconscious, and as noted, usually at least one side of it is beyond our level of consciousness. Our conflict follows us everywhere, and if not managed or balanced, it can cause great relationship difficulty. A couple decided to prematurely terminate couples therapy and spend their money on vacations. However, they could not seem to leave their conflict behind because I was told by their friends (also clients) that the couple were arguing all over the world. I have always said that an internalized conflict has a passport and visa; it goes where we go.

## Commitment and Conflict

While everyone has conflicts, one tends to loom larger than the rest, depending on the couple and their respective backgrounds. Some couples, for example, may have chronic conflicts about justice, success, or power (Betchen, 2010; Betchen & Davidson, 2018). In this book, I am focused specifically on couples who have a predominant conflict with romantic commitment. That is, when one part of each partner wants to make a commitment and the other part feels uncomfortable doing so. For example, if the part of you that desires to commit is dominating, you might try to commit to someone. But then the other part of you might prevent it or render the commitment short-lived.

Specifically, it may psychologically block you from attaching, achieving intimacy, or falling passionately in love, all of which are symptomatic of not fully committing yourself to your partner and the relationship.

If a conflict with commitment is unbalanced, it might be difficult if not impossible for the relationship to last. If partners agree on the level of commitment, their conflict in the context of attachment, love, intimacy, and passion is said to be balanced (see Figure 3.1). If they disagree, however, their conflict is said to be unbalanced. For example, one partner may desire more intimacy and passion than the other and thus unbalance their conflict (see Figure 3.2).

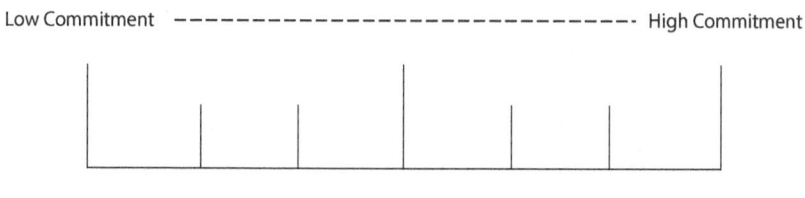

Couple Agrees on Level of Intimacy

*Figure 3.1* Balanced Commitment.

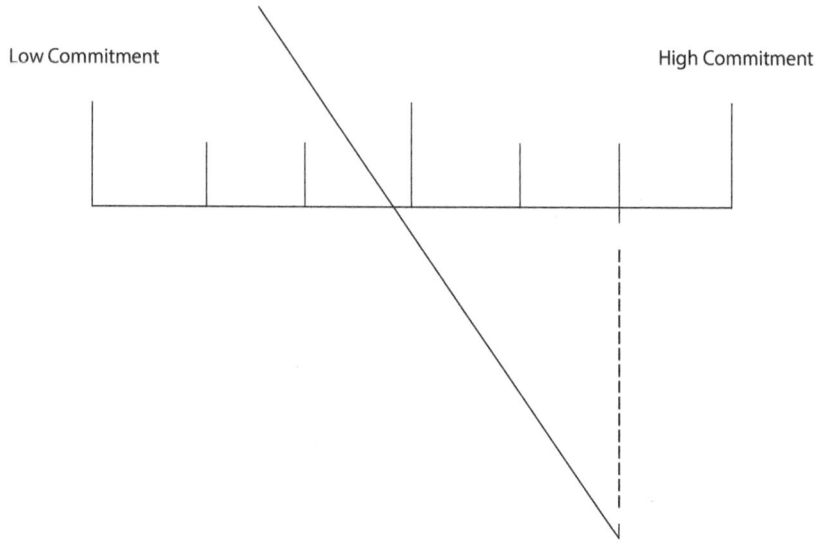

Couple Disagrees on Level of Intimacy

*Figure 3.2* Unbalanced Commitment.

As noted, while there are several conflicts – which vary in couples depending on their family of origin and life experiences – the focus here is on the *committed versus uncommitted* conflict. Internalized conflicts are difficult to control in part, because they are lodged in the unconscious.

The conscious part of the individual may try and battle it, not realizing that the unconscious side is putting up a fight. In fact, therapists will see an individual struggling to commit but with no history of successful commitment. No matter how hard this person might try, it is like witnessing a Sisyphean venture. Consider the following example.

Larry was a single 64-year-old man who presented for couples therapy with his Asian American (Chinese) fiancée, Amy. Larry had been engaged four times throughout his life, but each time marriage was close, he found some excuse to escape the commitment. In all fairness to Larry, some of the women he chose had significant problems of their own. For example, one woman was an alcoholic, another was bipolar who refused medical treatment, and one of them had very dysfunctional children from a previous marriage.

The pattern is clear – each of Larry's choices was designed to help him avoid the ultimate commitment of marriage. Sometimes he minimized his partners' problems, other times he was in complete denial, and other times he exacerbated them with controlling, selfish behavior. Nevertheless, as Larry aged, he could no longer adequately defend against the loneliness he experienced being on his own or the fear of aging alone. That is, the part of Larry that wanted to commit was slowly winning out over the side that wanted to avoid it.

Finding Amy, a younger, relatively docile woman was Larry's best chance to form a committed relationship. But it was obvious that he was having difficulty. While he could be a loving partner to Amy, he would forget her birthdays and other holidays important to her. He also made it difficult for her family to visit. Larry claimed that he loved Amy and was very attracted to her, yet his struggle was palpable. Amy's patience was beginning to wane.

The key to treatment success, as you will find out in Chapters 5 and 6, is to uncover the conflict with romantic commitment, determine its origin, and integrate both sides of the conflict to achieve a healthy, functional balance. Couples must get used to the fact that conflicts of this magnitude never completely dissipate. Clients only need attempt to expose, control, and manage them. In this sense there is no cure for an internal conflict, and so couples must expect a flare-up time and again.

## Shared Conflict

Clinicians find that when a couple presents for treatment, one of the partners appears less committed (like Larry) to the relationship while the other (like Amy) appears to pursue commitment (Stanley, 2016). But as mentioned, they share one thing in common: an underlying conflict with commitment – both want commitment but sabotage it albeit in different ways, as the less committed partner has a problem with committing and the committed partner has a problem with allowing him/herself to be committed to. Again, the symptoms may or may not be conscious to their respective partners, but the underlying commitment conflict tends to emanate from each partner's family of origin and dwell in their individual and collective unconscious. Consider the case of Lisa and Craig.

Lisa stopped having sex with her husband Craig for no apparent reason. She claimed that Craig was a very handsome, loving man who had always taken care of her, but that she was no longer interested in having sex with him. She had love for Craig, but her intimacy, passion, and commitment waned, and she admitted that she was not "in love" with him.

Craig was baffled but oddly did not question Lisa's commitment to their relationship. Instead, he continuously asked her if there was anything more that he could do for her; he was hanging onto the relationship as best he could.

As Lisa's treatment progressed, she was able to connect her chaotic and splintered family of origin (e.g., her father left when she was a teenager and her mother worked two jobs to pay the bills, often leaving Lisa and her younger sister to fend for themselves) to an internalized conflict with commitment: she felt both comfortable and uncomfortable being taken care of. She was happy and relieved to be rescued by Craig and his family but never felt comfortable being cared for. She used to say that although she enjoyed the closeness and supportive nature of Craig's big family, she felt like an "outsider." But even with this level of insight, Lisa did not see herself as having a conflict with commitment.

Craig's conflict with commitment was anchored in his need to rescue while being annoyed by the burden and lack of reciprocity that usually come with it. His conflict showed in taking the risk of marrying someone so young and needy, his rescuing of her, and his tolerating her lack of desire for him. The couple's shared conflict with commitment would put them both at the very low end of the romantic continuum and make it virtually impossible to ever achieve a durable romantic commitment.

As a general matter, individuals with the same conflict are drawn to one another just as Craig and Lisa were. The attraction is usually unconscious but nevertheless powerful. This is not to suggest that physical attraction is not a factor. I believe that individuals choose people they are attracted to emotionally and physically. But for the relationship to take hold, they must share a conflict. The choice process is usually unconscious but operates with great accuracy, especially as it is applied to long-term relationships and marriage.

While people searching for a sexual encounter or short-term relationship may be matched up via their mutual conflicts, this is not necessarily required. Anyone, for example, can be physically attracted to someone and have sex without the influence of a conflict. For the relationship to become significant, however, the conflicts play a major matchmaking role. But why is this so? What is the significance of selecting someone with the same conflict?

Creating a shared conflict first and foremost helps each partner to avoid the anxiety (unknown future) and depression (loss of the familiar) that often accompany change. It therefore preserves the familiar and the conflict. In this context, it maintains a conflict with romantic commitment.

While a conflict with commitment causes pain and brings the couple to therapy, it also protects both partners, counterintuitively, from a world they are unfamiliar with but offers hope that the relationship will be rescued from the brink. While this attraction is nearly always a choice influenced by each partner's family of origin, it helps to debunk the adage that "opposites attract" and supports the view that two partners unconsciously choose their "twin-in-conflict" (Betchen, 2010). Consider two more case examples.

John met Lucy in college and was instantly attracted to her, but she was no easy catch, forcing John to relentlessly pursue her. Once John was able to obtain a date with Lucy, however, she immediately warned him not to get too involved with her because she was considering moving across the country following graduation.

John was not deterred by Lucy's warning and believed strongly that her physical beauty and the fact that they had many shared interests made the pursuit worth it. After several dates, however, John began to realize that something deeper was connecting the two. Without knowing this before they began dating, it turned out that both he and Lucy were only children, parentified and severely triangulated by their parents in their respective families of origin. While both partners were surprised, they took it as a sign of a special bond. What they eventually discovered was this bond came with complications and that their similar pasts manifested in a conflict with commitment.

Lucy felt trapped by both her parents and extended family, which led to her ambivalence about getting too close to anyone for fear of being trapped again. This, in part, was why she warned John not to get too close at the onset of their dating process. And although John was wildly attracted to Lucy and remained so, he turned out to be a chronic cheater unable to commit fully to her. Eventually, the couple stopped dating and swore never to marry. The closest they could ever get to commitment was to serially cohabitate with others.

Renee met Hal in their senior year of college and dated without interruption until marriage. However, their relationship was fraught with fighting and cheating on Renee's part until she demanded they open their marriage. But even then, Renee would still break some of the rules of their arrangement. Renee decided to live with a lover three days a week and Hal was adamantly against this. In fact, Hal was against opening their marriage but feared Renee would leave him if he didn't.

Examining the pasts of each partner it was evident that as different as they looked, they shared a conflict with commitment; it simply manifested differently. Renee, for example, had her pick of men and cheated on whoever she was with. She would start out strong with a sense of excitement and passion but quickly got bored and began to see other people. Hal even told me that when he married Renee, he knew it would not be long before she would sleep with other men. But he married her anyway. He said she was wildly attractive and sexy, and he never imagined ever getting a woman like her to date him, let alone marry him. When the couple came for treatment, Hal was begging Renee to give up their open marriage and to learn how to commit to him. Renee, however, was resistant to the idea. She claimed that she liked the new man she was with too much to break off with him.

Renee was the youngest child of three siblings. She admitted that being the youngest she was spoiled in part, because her parents had more money when she was born, and they wanted to make up for what they could not give her older siblings. Renee was also blessed with good looks.

Renee saw her upbringing as wonderful, except for her mother's seemingly constant flirting with men, including Renee's teachers. This, according to Renee, caused her much embarrassment. She also felt sorry for her father who Renee believed was just satisfied being with his much more attractive wife.

The tipping point for Renee was when her mother began to have an affair with a wealthy neighbor. This enraged and disgusted Renee, but what upset her even more was her father knew about the affair and sat by passively. Given this background, Renee decided that although she detested her mother's behavior, she would never be vulnerable to a man. Renee would always have the power, even though this led to her internal conflict with romantic commitment.

Hal was attractive enough to date when he was a young man, but he generally did not have his pick of women. In fact, Hals's high school and early college girlfriends cheated on him even though he catered to them in every way. Despite friends and family cajoling Hal to break up with these women, he decided to put up with their infidelities.

Hal claimed he was the neglected middle sibling of four. He described his father and mother as narcissistic people who insisted on having their needs met no matter the cost to the children. For example, they would often go on trips together and leave the children at home alone. Hal said his oldest sibling was in charge but not happy about it and sometimes took his frustration out on Hal and his younger sibling.

While it looks like Hal and Renee were polar-opposites, Renee demonstrates her conflict with commitment by never being faithful to or intimate with Hal or any man for that matter. At times, she was even sadistic toward them. Hal demonstrated his conflict with commitment by his pleasing, masochistic contribution to his marriage.

## Underestimating Conflict

When couples present for therapy, most partners firmly believe they are having difficulty because of their differences. In the context of commitment, again the committed partner appears committed to the relationship, while the uncommitted partner looks as if he/she cannot wait to end the relationship and set themselves free.

Given the sharply distinct attitudes and behaviors presented to the couples therapist, it is easy to believe that difference is the issue; even the most skilled clinician could be swayed by this disparate interaction. I, however, have found this to be a potentially costly therapeutic miscalculation. It is clear by now that I believe that when one partner has low commitment, both partners do. While this complicates the treatment process, to see it otherwise could lead to an unbalancing of the treatment in favor of the seemingly committed partner, enable the committed partner to escape change, lose systemic perspective, and neglect an entire piece of the couple's puzzle, leading to a misdiagnosis of the couple and their true dynamic. The clinician must keep in mind that even the apparent seeker of commitment demonstrates low commitment by unconsciously enabling their counterpart's ambivalence. Again, both partners are in possession of an internal conflict with romantic commitment and seek each other out because of this very sameness.

A second miscalculation often made by couples and couples' therapists is that the couple's underlying conflict – in this case a conflict with commitment – is finally under control and therefore no longer a serious threat to the couple's relationship. It may certainly look this way. But if the conflict is still out of control, it could flare up at any time and become even more dangerous. Consider the following example.

A supervisee, Janice, presented with a female client in supervision, Gwen, who was admittedly a worrier. Gwen said that her way of controlling her anxiety was to try and maintain as much control over herself, her household and children, and her husband Ian. She routinely avoided placing herself in potentially dangerous situations, whether it be avoiding a ride on a roller coaster at a theme park or attending concerts with large crowds. She ate well, rarely drank, and exercised regularly.

Gwen applied these control tactics along with taking an anti-anxiety medication. Ironically, however, Gwen married a man with a history of cheating who continued his streak of infidelities after marrying her. But with approximately two years of therapy under their belts, Janice was convinced that the couple were settled and under control for the first time in years. She was proud of her work and optimistic about the future of the couple, and I can understand why.

Following his last fling, Ian continued to attend weekly sessions with Gwen, each had an individual therapist, and each attended decided to attend church together. Although the couple had made vast personal and relational improvements, and Janice did a great job, I was cautious because she did not present any evidence to me that the couple really understood their underlying conflict with commitment. Despite all the professionals involved in the case, I believed they could still easily lose control and become symptomatic at any given moment.

Ian committed to no one his entire life even though there were moments he had a chance. Was he really in charge of his conflict and able to fully commit to Gwen, or was he simply following orders and "selling" both Gwen and Janice that he could be a good boy? Was he really in love with Gwen or just interested in a home base from which to cheat – the best of both worlds? Did Gwen stop looking long enough at Ian's behavior to gain insight into why she chose a man like him when it was obvious that he had never had a successful relationship in his lifetime? And was she healthy enough to leave him if he reverted to his cheating ways? Given my trepidation I chose to push my supervisee to continue to work on the couple's conflict with commitment.

Some couples go out of their way to present themselves as a "perfect match." Their conflict with commitment may be completely out of control, but they try to hide it from the outside world. Consider the following cases.

Tom told his family physician that he was having marital trouble, but his doctor could not believe it. "I thought you and your wife had a perfect marriage," the doctor exclaimed. Tom, however, reported in couples therapy that going on a date with his wife Lucy was like "going by himself." When I asked him to elaborate, he said that Lucy was an aloof person who rarely interacted with him unless it had something to do with what she perceived as "important" such as finances or their children. In fact, Tom recently gave up on his favorite activity – going to a movie and discussing it over drinks afterward – claiming that his wife showed no interest. Although he said that Lucy was always aloof, her emotional distancing had increased over the years, and he now feels markedly lonely.

What was particularly interesting about Tom and Lucy is that they were married for many years, not engaged in many overt altercations, and their sex life was rated by both partners as quite satisfying. Lucy even claimed to be happy with the marriage. Her response to Tom's accusations was that she was not an outgoing person and detested small talk. But as Lucy's emotional ambivalence grew stronger, she one day asked Tom for a divorce. She claimed that she had fallen in love with a man at work and was moving on. Tom and Lucy's relationship was void of romantic commitment for some time, and Lucy's aloof behavior was a sign.

A second example is that of a woman, Sarah, who, despite portraying herself to the outside world as having the perfect marriage, admitted to her husband, Lee, in couples therapy that she was never emotionally or romantically committed to their relationship. When I asked her why she married, she said that she had a "checklist" of what she wanted in a man and Lee met all the criteria at the time: he was a loyal, a good provider, and she knew he would make a great father. But soon Sarah stopped having sex with Lee and even found it hard to kiss him. The couple met in church and Sarah said that she was raised to marry someone within her faith without concern for physical attraction and passion. Lee not only met Sarah's requirements, but he was also handsome and adoring. But Sarah was ambivalent from the start and finally ended their relationship soon after they had their third and last child.

And last, within a year of Tim's divorce, he began dating a woman, Katie, whom he found extremely attractive. The couple shared good times together and had great sex. But Tim failed to introduce Katie to his friends and family, especially the two children he had with his ex-wife. In couples therapy Katie expressed concern about being separate from Tim's extended family life, but Tim offered no answers. After ten months of dating, however, Tim admitted to Katie that he was trying to hold onto the relationship but at a distance because he did not think it had a future. His main reason was that he did not think she would be a good enough stepmother to his children. Tim made this decision several months ago but was not ready to end the relationship.

Sensing Tim's ambivalence about deepening the relationship, Katie feared that if she pressed the issue, she would lose him. She, in fact, knew that Tim was not fully committed to their relationship, but she did not know why. When Tim told Katie the truth, she was heartbroken, and the couple dissolved their relationship.

## References

Bennett, K. (2023, June). The 3 worst fears about winning the lottery: After the reality of winning sinks in, watch out for these changes. *Psychology Today*. https://www.psychologytoday.com/us/blog/modern-minds/202306/the-3-worst-fears-about-winning-the-lottery

Betchen, S. (2010). *Magnetic partners: Discover how the hidden conflict that once attracted you to each other is now driving you apart*. Free Press.

Betchen, S., & Davidson, H. (2018). *Master conflict therapy: A new model for practicing couples and sex therapy*. Routledge.

Lindqvist, E., Östling, R., & Cesarini, D. (2020). Long-run effects of lottery wealth on psychological well-being. *Review of Economic Studies, 87*, 2703–2726. https://doi.org/10.1093/rstud/rdaa006

Stanley, S. M. (2016, November). What happens when partners aren't equally committed: New study examines relationships where one is just not into the other. *Psychology Today*. https://www.psychologytoday.com/us/blog/sliding-vs-deciding/201611/what-happens-when-partners-arent-equally-committed

# Chapter 4

# The Origin of the Romantic Committed and Uncommitted

Jamison and Lo (2020) wrote:

> Important decisions about romantic relationships are often made during adulthood, but the foundations for healthy relationships begin during childhood. Romantic development is related to experiences in the family of origin such as parenting, parents' romantic history, and patterns of interaction within families.
>
> (p. 84)

Runcan et al. (2012) wrote: "Communication is the engine of social relationships and upon it depend the quality of relationship or its bankruptcy" (p. 904)! The authors also said that communication is the process of sending one's ideas, information, emotions, and feelings to another person. They break communication down into three levels: logic is only responsible for approximately 7% of communicating; paraverbal (tone and volume) makes up 38%; and nonverbal (facial signs and body posture) accounts for 55%. The authors reported if there is no contradiction or confusion in these messages, communication can be an effective tool in relationships.

Verbal messages from a parent can leave a lasting impression on a child. Writing for the Center for Effective Parenting, Zolten and Long (2006) claimed that "children begin to form ideas and beliefs about themselves based on how their parents communicate with them" (p. 1). I have found that parents are surprised when their child quotes them after years. These same parents tell me they did not think their child paid any attention to what they said.

Those who appear romantically committed in treatment also have been influenced by certain messages and behaviors transmitted to them by their families of origin. In my experience, four major vehicles of communication – verbal messages, nonverbal cues and signals, behaviors witnessed, and family dynamics – serve to transmit these messages, which, in turn, may help to develop an internalized conflict with commitment capable of impacting their adult romantic relationships.

DOI: 10.4324/9781003475743-5

## The Committed

### Verbal Messages

Liz was the middle child of four. Her father had a bad temper and would drink every day after work until he got drunk. He would then start a fight and pass out for the night. While her older sister challenged her father's irresponsible and reckless behavior, Liz hid in her bedroom or took solace at a friend's house to avoid her father's wrath. In her teenage years, Liz became more knowledgeable about alcoholism and abuse and would confront her passive mother about her enabling. She told her mother to either set limits with her father or leave him. But her mother offered a telling response: "Liz, you will amount to nothing in life if you quit during hard times."

Liz was in conflict. She thought her mother was pathetic and self-sacrificing for allowing her father's behavior to continue and swore to herself that she would not follow in kind when she chose a mate. But in explaining why she put up with his antics to her children, she presented the same mantra her mother had given her: "Don't be a quitter."

### Nonverbal Cues and Signals

Even if Diana did not receive the direct message to "never quit" like Liz did, she received nonverbal cues that likely contributed to her conflict with commitment. Diana studied ballet from childhood until her 20s. Her mother had always wanted to be a professional ballerina and made it into a big company for a short time before a career-ending injury forced her to retire. When Diana was born, her mother saw it as an opportunity to make up for her misfortune by encouraging Diana to take up ballet. Diana wanted to please her mother and took years of lessons. But as the competition grew and the need to give more of her life to ballet, Diana grew tired. She was also frustrated with the constant need to watch her weight.

In her late twenties, Diana finally freed herself and gave up ballet. But from that point onward, her mother barely spoke to her and would leave a room in the middle of her sentences. Diana claimed that her mother was so disappointed with her that she shunned her. Diana said:

> We still do not speak unless there is a family emergency. I believe she is so enraged with me for ruining her dream that she cannot even talk about it. Shutting down like this is her way of punishing someone. And now that someone is me.

Although Diana reported that her relationship with her mother caused her pain, when she reported for treatment with her husband, Rob, she was shunning him for quitting a job that he hated. She also withdrew sex. Rob reported that he was literally scared to upset Diana for fear of her shutting down. He added that this interfered with intimacy in their relationship because he is afraid to disagree with her or talk to her about anything controversial. "I just don't know what will trigger her, but her shunning can last for weeks. She is a grudge holder like her mother," he said.

Diana was in conflict. She was conscious of her tendency to replicate her mother's grudge-holding behavior – the type of behavior that she once found so painful. But she also knew it was a very effective punishment that she could use to make her point without verbalizing it.

### Behaviors Witnessed

The cases of Liz and Diana beg the question: How could both women replicate their respective mothers' enabling behaviors when it caused them so much pain in their childhoods? My response is that both received strong verbal and nonverbal messages, respectively, from their mothers. But they also "witnessed" behaviors not favorable to role modeling romantic commitment. This consistent level of reinforcement made it likely that Liz and Diana would have difficulty in adult romantic relationships.

It is quite common for children like Liz and Diana to experience more than one of the influential messages simultaneously in their families of origin. Some, unfortunately, experience all four messages, which will almost guarantee an unbalanced conflict with commitment in their adult relationships. The greater number of messages conveyed and their consistency, as well as their level of intensity, the more easily they will make an impression on the child that will be internalized and transmitted to adulthood relationships.

### Family Dynamics

The committed can also be highly influenced by becoming enlisted in their respective family dynamics. Direct involvement or playing an active role in family interactions holds perhaps the most power over the child and can follow them well into adulthood. Consider the following example.

Harold was the youngest child of three siblings. But the age gap was so great between them all that he was essentially raised like an only child. Harold's parents fought frequently, mostly about money, and each parent would often complain about the other to Harold. Harold heard from his mother that his father was lazy and stubborn and his father that his mother's expectations were unreasonable.

Harold experienced many sleepless nights listening to his parents' fights. And when they weren't fighting, they would sometimes refrain from speaking to each other for weeks at a time. Harold's parents reinforced his mediation role by repeatedly telling him that they would not know what to do without him. He therefore got both verbal and nonverbal messages that he was to mediate his parents' marriage. He also witnessed their fighting first-hand, which served to actively enlist him in his parents' dynamics. Blaisure and Saposnek (2023), writing for the American Association for Marriage and Family Therapy, claimed that putting children in the mediating position by asking them to carry messages between parents is especially detrimental to the children.

When I met Harold, he and his wife, June, were fighting furiously over Harold's inability to set limits with his parents – he was still mediating. But what was readily noticeable was how loyal Harold was not only to his parents but also to his wife that seemed void of any kind of empathy or ability to compromise.

June was a highly demanding, controlling woman. And Harold wanted to please her but not at the expense of his parents. Rather, Harold desperately tried to commit equal time to his wife and parents, but rather than challenge all of them on their needy and demanding behavior, he continued to loyally toil away.

## The Uncommitted

### Verbal Messages

If a parent happens to send a message criticizing or belittling romantic commitment, consciously or unconsciously, it could impact the child's future perception of relationship commitment or create a conflict in this area. In most cases, I do not believe that something said once will necessarily follow a child into adulthood. But if the same message is conveyed over time, it may have an influence. Consider the following examples.

From the time Bill could remember, his father told him not to commit to a woman until he had completed all his education and settled into a career. He said women were "trouble" and would "ruin" Bill's life. He said the primary reason for this was because "women are never satisfied." Bill's father further explained that once Bill got into a relationship with a woman, he would be limited by her needs and desires and not be free to achieve professionally.

With this message deeply ingrained, Bill graduated from college and had the drive and tenacity to pursue a foreign medical degree – the only medical school he was accepted to at the time. When asked how he enjoyed the country he was studying in, Bill said that he did not take the time to see the sights around or to date any women. He said his goal was to become a doctor and he had no interest in anything else.

Once Bill graduated from medical school and completed his residency, he pursued fellowship after fellowship until he was in his early 40s. It was not until he was exhausted from all the schooling that he finally entertained the idea of committing to someone. After meeting a nurse, Sally, at a hospital he was working at, he tried to be exclusive but had little time for her as he then pursued promotion after promotion. Sally reported that the relationship was passionless and void of intimacy because Bill was preoccupied with achievement. This is the reason she insisted on couples therapy.

Although Bill struggled to put off his academic pursuits to attend sessions, he managed to do so. And while he was defensive in treatment, Bill was eventually able to admit that he had been in conflict over his father's message for many years. He said that although he was proud of his accomplishments, he was a lonely man who longed to marry and have a family. He also said that he loved his father very much but came to realize that his father was not completely objective. He explained that his father was unhappy with his own achievements and had blamed his limitations on Bill's mother. Bill was in conflict. He took his father's message to heart about staying away from women because he did not want to let his father down – he claimed that his achievements made his father happy. But he also longed to marry and start a family.

Gina was the oldest of two daughters in a single-parent household. Her father had left her mother soon after Gina's little sister was born. Times were tough financially, and Gina's mother worked two jobs to support herself and her daughters. She saw her situation as quite unfair given that her estranged husband earned a lucrative income. Gina's mother, in a tone of anger and disgust, regularly gave both daughters the verbal message that men cannot be counted on. "They will let you down when you need them the most," she would say. Gina missed her father, but when he eventually re-appeared and tried to be a part of her life, Gina's mother made it a difficult process and continued to ridicule him.

Gina admittedly grew up fearful and distrusting of men. She did have a series of relationships in her adult life but would find a way to end them before they went too far. Tellingly, Gina was engaged a total of three times, and each time she would back out before the relationship deepened. There was little passion in these relationships, in part because she was fearful of becoming pregnant. She also never achieved an orgasm with a man and admitted that she experienced anxiety the closer she got to commitment.

However, there was evidence that Gina was in conflict. She never gave up looking for love, and when I first met her, she was in a relatively long-term relationship with her boyfriend, Troy. She said that she really liked Troy and wanted to trust him, but she was having difficulty. She also said that she was tired of being asked about her relationship status by friends and relatives. She said she felt like a "loser." Gina had "a desire to be considered normal" – she wanted to "trust" men and to improve her low self-esteem.

### Nonverbal Cues and Signals

Burgoon et al. (2021) wrote: "Nonverbal messages color the meanings of interpersonal relationships. Humans rely on facial, head, postural, and vocal signals to express relational messages along continua" (p. 1). These messages are often more subtle than verbal messages but nevertheless can have a powerful impact (Dunbar & Bernhold, 2019). And it is not that difficult for a child or teenager to figure out that a parent is dissatisfied. Consider the following example.

When Nick was young, he and his father would take car drives in the country quite frequently but rarely spoke. His father was an old-school, tough guy who did not believe in small talk, but he seemed to enjoy the peacefulness of nature and he liked having Nick with him. Nick, however, was needy. He looked at these rides as an opportunity to connect with his father and get some fatherly advice about life. But each time Nick would try to engage, his father would not respond. Nick said he would just sit in silence or just grunt. Nick said it was as if his father was in his own world.

Nick added that if he asked whether his father was annoyed about something, his father would wave his hand in a dismissive manner. He said it was his father's way of saying the discussion was not worth the effort or whatever Nick was considering was a bad idea. For example, every time Nick spoke about a specific girl he liked, his father would only frown and wave his hand. Nick's interpretation of this was that his father was telling him that women were not worth the trouble. Nick truly believed that his father saw women as impossible to satisfy and that relationships were doomed.

Nonetheless, Nick had sex with a lot of women. But when it came to commitment, he shied away. While he would not model the nonverbal messages his father did, he would echo them by openly complaining that women were controlling and impossible to please. His main mantra was that women were an "annoying species."

In couple's treatment, my experience with nonverbal messages between partners usually comes in the form of an eye roll, a frown, an exasperated sigh, a shift in body posture away from each other, or a dismissive wave of the hand. By the time Nick sought me out for couples therapy, thanks to some individual therapy, he had become more objective about women, and to his credit, in a somewhat stable relationship with a divorcee, Erin.

Erin complained that Nick often dismissed her with eye rolling and sighs and that her marriage was completely void of intimacy. She said she felt Nick did not love her but was with her out of convenience – as in a transactional relationship. Erin claimed the couple did have passionate sex when Nick felt the need, but immediately afterward, he would either fall asleep or jump out of bed, shower, and go about his business.

Nick realized that this might be his last chance to marry, and he did not want to lose Erin. He admitted that he was in conflict: while he stuck to his plan to keep women at a distance, he also claimed that as he aged, he feared if he did not fix his problem he would die alone. Nick also found sex with random women somewhat "boring," and he felt the women he was with were using him as much as he used them. Nick knew that he was not being objective about women. But he worked to overcome his trust issues and his need to protect himself from romantic commitment with the use of distance.

While parents may communicate both verbal and nonverbal messages simultaneously, perhaps an even more potent way of transmitting anti-commitment messages to children is to demonstrate a low commitment so that the children can see it firsthand.

### Behaviors Witnessed

Children do not have to become directly engaged with their parents to internalize a conflict with commitment. In fact, they are heavily influenced by the actions of their parents just by witnessing their behavior toward one another. Consider the following example.

Caitlin presented for couples work with her boyfriend, Todd, because of constant fighting. Todd claimed that Caitlin consistently ridiculed him but seemed to take special satisfaction in emasculating him in front of other men. Todd said that he rarely challenged Caitlin, but he asked her many times in private if she could save her anger until they were alone, but she refused. Todd insisted that if he confronted Caitlin about anything, it would only make her angrier and more verbally abusive. It was interesting to note that in treatment Todd always referred to his wife as "dear," while Caitlin would call Todd names such as "loser" or "idiot." Caitlin took no responsibility for her poor treatment of Todd, claiming that he deserved it.

Caitlin had a history of abusing men, and she would do so until she got bored of them. Caitlin said that she was always in charge in her relationships and that no man had ever broken up with her. Working with Caitlin in treatment was challenging, but she eventually felt comfortable enough to say that she often witnessed her father verbally abusing her mother. "It didn't matter where we were, my dad always found something to use to embarrass mom," she said, "and my mom could not seem to defend herself." Apparently, her mother's main coping skill was to make a joke out of the situation to diffuse it to spare public embarrassment. When asked what role she played in this dynamic, Caitlin said that her older sister took her father on, but she hid in her bedroom or stayed with friends. She said that as soon as her father pulled his car in the driveway, she "disappeared."

Although Caitlin felt powerless as a child, she later sadistically took her rage out on the men she dated. She also happened to have an uncanny radar for finding masochistic men to tolerate her abuse, and Todd was one such man. But Caitlin also said that if she truly hated men, she would not date as often as she did.

Caitlin was in conflict. She took her sadistic rage for her father out on the men who were masochistic, but she longed for a stable relationship with one. She said it was better to be the abuser than the abused. She was in treatment because she thought Todd was worth the effort.

Geri described her mother as "passive and infantile" and her father as distant. She claimed that her father would sometimes leave home for a month at a time. She suspected him of having affairs, but she could never substantiate this. Geri loved her father but felt that he preferred other women over her, and this affected her self-esteem. When Geri sensed that her father was about to leave home, she would cry hysterically and beg him to stay, but he would still go. She also witnessed her mother's inability to set limits with him – apparently, she would always take him back no matter how long he was away.

From observing her father's distancing and her mother's powerlessness, Geri had difficulty trusting men. She claimed that they were too dangerous to show vulnerability to. She also saw herself as "less than" and powerless to hold a man and to make him love her. To cope with these perceptions, Geri kept her "distance" from men as best she could. When she did get into a relationship, she demanded more than they could give her, forcing them to abandon her. Geri was in conflict: she wanted to be loved but did not feel she deserved to be, and she was too afraid to seriously commit to anyone over the long term.

### Family Dynamics

As noted, some children are directly engaged in the family dynamics and are more vulnerable to developing and internalizing a conflict with romantic commitment. Writing from a psychoanalytic perspective, Schmideberg (1948) noted that deprived parents may unconsciously treat their children as parental figures. But two systems therapists are perhaps most closely associated with the dynamic. Minuchin et al. (1967) called juvenile delinquents who were given adult-oriented tasks such as child-rearing "parental children." Bozsormenyi-Nagy (1965) coined the term *parentification* to indicate when a child is given age-inappropriate responsibilities. Most commonly the child becomes the parent and the parents become the children. Parentified children are usually considered the most competent and able to do what is needed to keep the family functioning.

Parentified children are often the child of infantile parents, sick or elderly parents, the child of single-parents, or the child of at least incompetent or overwhelmed parents. Whatever the reason, the parentified child is tasked with the enormous responsibility to master an impossible job and with little to no resources. It is no reason why many are skeptical of commitment in adulthood. Consider the following example of a parentified woman who refused to commit to anyone for fear of being re-parentified.

Roberta was the oldest daughter of six siblings. Both her father and mother were alcoholics who worked at the same factory. After work every day, they would stop at the neighborhood bar, get drunk, and stay until it closed in the evening. Sometimes they were in no shape to walk home, and Roberta would have to pick them up. Roberta claimed that her parents slept late on weekends because of hangovers and rarely took care of their children. Roberta made all the meals, attended parent–teacher conferences, and made sure her siblings took baths and dressed appropriately. Although her parents made enough money together to sustain the family financially, they had no idea how to take care of their money, and so Roberta kept the books and allotted enough money to care for her siblings.

Roberta did not see any point in complaining to her parents, so she accepted her position with a somewhat fatalistic attitude. She had no social life and no time to date in her teenage years. She reported that she longed to have her own life but felt bad for her younger siblings and considered it her obligation to care for them.

As an adult, Roberta kept a great "distance" from men for fear of getting trapped into marriage. She believed that whoever she committed to would want children and she had no energy left to raise her own babies. Roberta never had time to go to college when she was caretaking her family, but in her later years, she made it a priority to complete a two-year nursing program. While in nursing school, she was introduced to a young medical student, Greg, whom she found very attractive. This is when Roberta decided to seek counseling. Her conflict with commitment was that she wanted to feel comfortable with Greg and be "normal" for the first time in her life, but the fear of being trapped blocked her.

Joan's parents constantly told her how smart she was and how far she would go in life if she applied herself. They also told her that if she kept her grades up, they would do anything in their power to support her and to help make her dreams come true. Joan was an excellent student and longed to be a doctor. After getting into a prestigious college that only offered a partial scholarship, Joan went to her parents for the support they had previously promised but was shocked when they laughed at her and said that they had changed their mind about college. They no longer saw it as a sound investment.

Joan was not surprised that her mother took this attitude, but she was stunned by her father's reaction. She had always trusted him and his promises of support. With this traumatic experience, Joan began to look more closely at some of her father's other promises and began to see him as a manipulative liar. Working two jobs, Joan got herself through community college and a four-year university, albeit both were beneath her academic ability. Disheartened, she took a job as a computer programmer in a mid-size company and made it her life's career.

Joan met Ed at her company. Ed was an engineer and the two immediately connected. However, once they began dating, Joan kept a close watch on Ed. She followed his every word for inconsistencies, checked his cell phone and computer when he wasn't watching, and proved to be jealous of every woman he spoke to, even colleagues. Exasperated, Ed begged Joan to attend couples therapy. Joan was in conflict: she loved Ed and wanted to move in with him but could not "trust" him even though he gave her no reason to distrust him. Joan was so traumatized by her parents' deceit that she could no longer trust anyone close to her, especially someone she believed she loved.

One way or another, our adult romantic relationships are influenced by our childhood experiences. Strebe (2023) believed that how we give and receive in a relationship are greatly influenced by one or both parents. The cases of Roberta and Joan support this point.

## References

Blaisure, K., & Saposnek, D. T. (2023). Managing conflict during divorce. *AAMFT* https://www.aamft.org/consumer_updates/managing_conflict_during_divorce.aspx?websitekey=8e8c9bd6-0b71-4cd1-a5ab-013b51855b01

Boszormenyi-Nagy, I. (1965). A theory of relationships: Experience and Transactions. In I. Boszormenyi-Nagy & J. Framo (Eds.), *Intensive family therapy: Theoretical and practical aspects* (pp. 33–86). Harper & Row.

Burgoon, J. K., Wang, X., Chen, X., Pentland, S. J., & Dunbar, N. E. (2021). Nonverbal behaviors "speak" relational messages of dominance, trust, and composure. *Frontiers in Psychology, 12*, 1–17. https://doi.org/10.3389/fpsyg.2021.624177

Dunbar, N. E., & Bernhold, Q. (2019). Interpersonal power and nonverbal communication. In C. R. Agnew and J. J. Harman (Eds.), *Power in close relationships: Interpersonal contexts* (pp. 261–278). Cambridge University Press.

Jamison, T. B., & Lo, H. Y. (2020). Exploring parents' ongoing role in romantic development: Insights from young adults. *Journal of Social and Personal Relationships, 38*, 84–102. https://doi.org/10.1177/0265407520958475

Minuchin, S., Montalvo, B., Guerney, B. G., Roseman, B., & Schumer, F. (1967). *Families of the slum*. Basic Books.

Runcan, P. L., Constantineanu, C., Ielics, B., & Popa, D. (2012). The role of communication in the parent-child interaction. *Procedia – Social and Behavioral Sciences, 46*, 904–908. https://doi.org/10.1016/j.sbspro.2012.05.221

Schmideberg, M. (1948). Parents as children. *Psychiatric Quarterly* Supplement, *22*, 207–218.

Strebe, S. (2023, August). Yes, your parents affect your future relationships – Here's how. *Brides*. https://www.brides.com/relationships-with-parents-5112051

Zolten, K., & Long, N. (2006). *Parent/child interaction*. Center for Effective Parenting. University of Arkansas for Medical Sciences. www.parenting-ed.org

# Clinical Assessment of Romantic Commitment

# Chapter 5

# Assessing Couples with Commitment Conflicts

Balderama-Durbin et al. (2016) claimed that "understanding couple distress requires that assessment extend beyond individual factors to include the broader relational and socioecological context" (p. 131). Ritchie et al. (2019) wrote:

> Assessment in couple and family therapy refers to the process by which a therapist evaluates the clients' individual and dyadic characteristics, and environmental circumstances. Clinical assessment is aimed at evaluating the nature, scope, and severity of the presenting concerns. It also includes collecting relevant information that may assist in selecting an appropriate course of treatment.
>
> (p. 144)

In my opinion, an accurate assessment is vital to the treatment success in part, because like many other things in life, "the way something begins, is the way it ends." Couples can be particularly chaotic and complex. If the initial assessment process is inadequate, it may lead the therapist and couple on an unproductive or harmful treatment path. The following example is that of a couple who, because of an incomplete assessment and poor diagnosis, suffered further hardship.

Mary and Al were a couple in their early 50s. The couple presented with Mary's pain during intercourse. Mary's discomfort proved to be quite a mystery for various therapists, psychiatrists, and pelvic floor specialists. She even had surgery, but this did not alleviate her pain. When I completed a full assessment on the couple, however, I determined that Mary suffered from low sexual desire that was related to an underlying conflict she had struggled with her entire life. That is, Mary was severely parentified as a child and developed "pleasure inhibition" as a result. Only when Mary began to examine her conflict with pleasure did her symptoms begin to dissipate.

DOI: 10.4324/9781003475743-7

Couples and students have often asked me why I attach such importance to a couple's pattern of interaction and why do I ask certain questions of a couple some of which seem completely unrelated to what the couple might have presented as their chief complaint. My response is that every interaction and every question I ask is aimed at ascertaining a couple's commitment to the treatment process, what their specific symptoms are, whether they have a shared conflict with commitment, and what is the best way to set up their treatment. Sometimes a direct question might only be met with a defense, and so it is important to ask several peripheral questions to work around these defenses and to help the couple to see the scope and magnitude of their internalized conflict with commitment.

As noted, it is believed that couples have a shared underlying conflict with commitment (i.e., they need it and yet avoid it), born out of each partner's respective families of origin. This conflict serves as an unconscious matchmaking device – partners are magnetically attracted to those with the same conflict and are compelled to bond. Once the couple is formed, it then operates as a formidable interactional collusion, with one partner playing the role of the committed and the other playing the role of the uncommitted. The objective is to protect the conflict so that each partner can avoid anxiety and other pain that might come with change.

When a couple's conflict is "optimally" balanced, the couple possess all the ingredients (i.e., attachment, love, passion, intimacy) of commitment, just enough of them, or an acceptable combination of them to satisfy both partners. The couple are then free of symptoms associated with these ingredients and considered to have a relatively durable relationship. If, however, the couple's conflict is unbalanced for too long a time, it means that one of or more of the key ingredients are missing or too low for at least one partner to tolerate. The couple will then exhibit significant symptoms in the context of the ingredients, thus putting the relationship at risk.

The objective of this model is to uncover the unconscious shared conflict with commitment, determine its origin and how it manifests in each partner – which partner assumes the role of the committed and which plays the role of the uncommitted – and help rebalance the conflict and alleviate any symptoms. Not all relationships survive this process. The couples therapist should not try to enable an abusive or tenuous relationship but rather help the couple do their best to establish a strong relationship. Hopefully, all the data gathered during the assessment process will offer the couples therapist a framework from which to work more efficiently and improve a couple's durability (see Figure 5.1).

## Initial Contact

Assessment of a conflict with commitment begins with the first contact that occurs usually between one partner and the therapist. While this contact is generally made by telephone or email, the therapist should be alert to signs

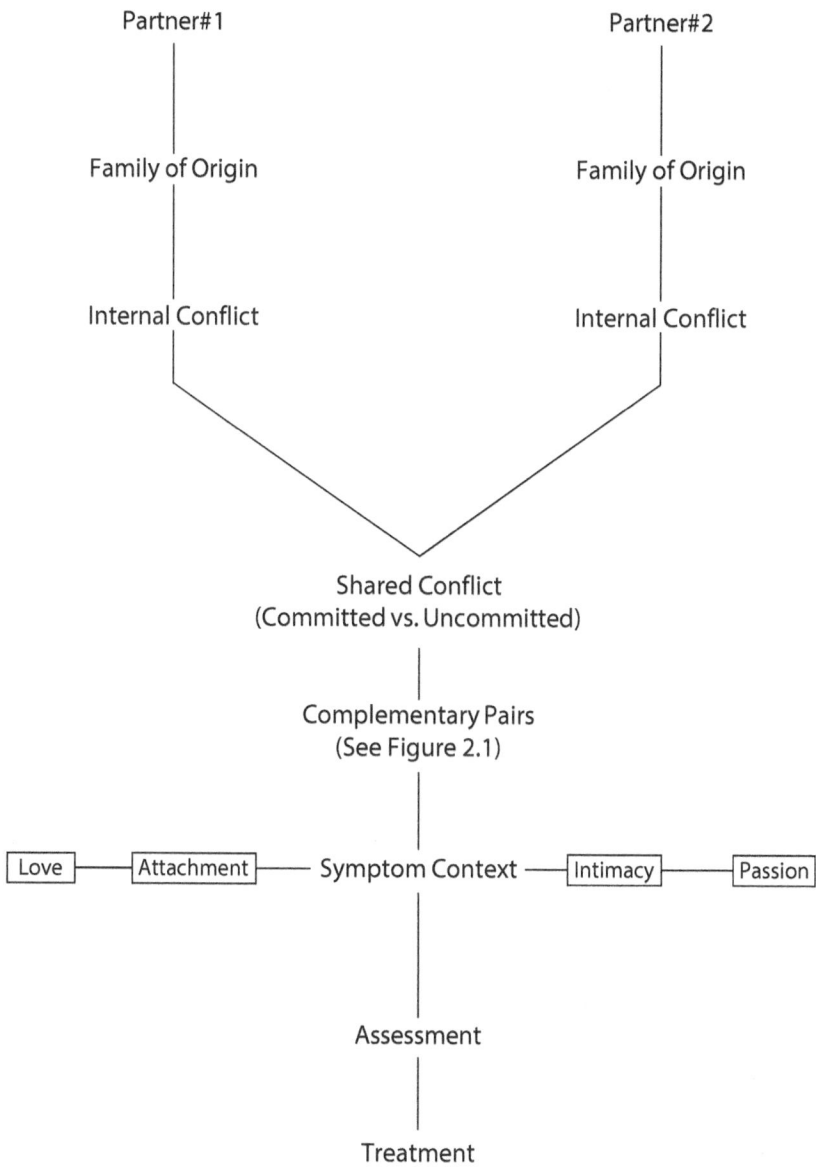

*Figure 5.1* Assessment Process.

that a couple is ambivalent about investing in treatment. The symptoms a couple present may be obvious, but more evidence will be needed to determine if there is an underlying conflict with commitment.

Doherty et al. (2021) found that from the onset of their problems, couples wait 2.68 years before seeking therapy. Although this is a far cry from the six years reported by The Gottman Institute (Gaspard, 2024), both agree that for the best outcome, it is important that both partners are invested in the treatment process. I do not offer any appointments until I can determine the couple's commitment to treatment. And one of the best ways to start this process is to simply ask.

Because it is usually the more invested partner who makes initial contact, you will most likely get an honest answer. Strauss-Cohen (2023) contended that it is the most uncomfortable partner who initiates treatment, not necessarily the most dysfunctional partner. In fact, the initiator tends to be the mover and shaker of the relationship. Some of these individuals have a proclivity to help others and to problem-solve. Speaking directly to the initiator makes it easier to determine whether their case is appropriate for my practice and to help determine how committed both partners are to treatment.

This does not, however, mean that the caller is always the most committed partner. Some who plan to separate or divorce, or as Winston (2018) put it are, "out the door," are simply looking for a therapist to take over and facilitate the process. This is especially true if they perceive their partner as infantile or, worse, suicidal.

Others may initiate a call under duress from their partner. For example, a female client threatened to have affairs with other men if her husband did not seek treatment for his sexual problem. And a male client refused to end his affair if his wife did not agree to go to couples therapy with him. He believed that his wife was so controlling and obstinate that the only way to save the marriage was to force her under extreme circumstances to go to therapy with him. Once she agreed, he stayed true to his word and ended his affair almost immediately.

In place of, or in conjunction with a live assessment, some therapists might send the couple a questionnaire or instrument to be completed prior to the first formal session. This tool may be useful in evaluating romantic commitment. Some instruments used include *The Relationship Commitment* Scale (Wiley et al., 2005), a scale suitable for both business and couples. This scale consists of four items on a five-point Likert Scale to measure commitment.

*The Relationship Assessment Scale* was developed by Hendrick et al. (1998) to measure global relationship satisfaction. The scale consists of seven items, each rated on a five-point Likert Scale. One of the seven items measured is "commitment." *The Enhanced Gottman Relationship Checkup* is an assessment tool consisting of five sections: (1) Friendship and Intimacy (e.g., relationship satisfaction, emotional connection, and romance); (2) The Safety Scales (e.g., trust, chaos, and commitment); (3) The Conflict Scales (e.g., stress and conflict management); (4) The Shared Meaning

System (e.g., values and goals); and (5) Individual Areas of Concern (e.g., individual issues such as sex, depression, and substance use) (Gottman & Gottman, 2024).

While various assessment scales can be helpful to both therapist and couple, the model used herein is based on my conflict theory model, a psychoanalytic/psychodynamic systems approach, which is less amenable to measurement (Betchen, 2010, 2022, 2024; Betchen & Davidson, 2018). And while a couple's symptoms are important in my approach, the main objective is to uncover the couple's shared, unconscious conflict with commitment. This, in itself, requires a live, spontaneous assessment where the therapist's intuitive skill and clinical experience are most valuable.

The assessment tool used in my model is the genogram (Bowen, 1978; DeMaria et al., 2017; Gambescia et al., 2021). The genogram is an instrument used to gather data about each partner, past and present, and to determine if any patterns exist that might be contributing to current symptoms. I use it primarily to track and connect each partner's symptoms to conflicts with commitment. I will discuss the genogram in more detail later in this chapter.

## Treatment Structure

If the caller is motivated to seek treatment, whether under duress or not, and agrees to abide by the structure of the treatment process, including following the rules regarding fees and missed appointments and filling out certain forms (e.g., consent to treat, permission forms to obtain or release case information), there is some room for optimism (Doherty, 2002; Weeks & Fife, 2014). If, however, the caller is hesitant to commit and sounds ambivalent about treatment; complains about the fee, the appointment time, and my model of treatment; demands special treatment; plays telephone tag with me for an inordinate amount of time (e.g., three weeks or more); or prevents the absent partner from attending sessions, an unbalanced conflict with commitment is likely to be operating.

Nevertheless, early resistance should be expected given that making a commitment to the treatment process often mirrors the couple's difficulty with making a commitment to the relationship; it also includes the task of choosing one side of the conflict over the other. Consider the following example of an initiating partner blocking a counterpart from attending sessions.

Sydney called me to set up a conjoint appointment with her and her boyfriend, Charlie. Sydney said she had been dating Charlie for eight years and, unlike him, she was ready to marry. According to Sydney, Charlie preferred to continue in an exclusive relationship with her while living together. Charlie's philosophy: "marriage is a paper contract that isn't needed if two people love each other."

Charlie's stance on marriage matched his skepticism about therapy. He rejected the notion that an outsider could instruct two people in love how to live their lives. Despite the resistance, however, Sydney assured me that Charlie would join her for treatment. Ironically, however, it was she who always seemed to find an excuse for Charlie's absence. Sydney would routinely ask for more individual sessions, claiming that she had to process her anger for Charlie. She would frequently tell me that Charlie was too busy with work to attend treatment or too sick. It was also common for a fight to break out just before a scheduled conjoint session that enabled one or both partners to refuse to attend the session. Sydney was the catalyst for these disruptions.

After assessing the initiating caller's interest in treatment, I ask whether their counterpart is willing to attend sessions. If the answer is "yes," it might be a sign that the couple are serious about getting help. It might also indicate that neither the caller nor the absent partner is sabotaging the onset of treatment. If the caller claims the counterpart is not interested in attending conjoint sessions, the case can still be workable but might be more challenging. In this sense, the couple would fit the typical combination of a seemingly committed partner and an uncommitted partner I mentioned earlier. This does not yet tell the therapist which partner is which but only that the combination exists in some form.

The general structure offered in this model is to preferably see the couple together in the first and second sessions to allow for the full assessment. These sessions are then followed by two individual sessions – one for each partner. I give the initiator this information in our first contact.

Scholars have long debated the appropriateness of conducting individual sessions in the context of couples therapy. Berman (1982) saw the value in allowing a limited number of individual sessions in conjoint treatment. She claimed the main reason for this is to resolve any therapeutic blocks in the treatment process such as when important information is being withheld. Leone (2023), writing from a psychoanalytic perspective, claimed that individual sessions "can be an attuned, empathic response to the needs of one or both partners and the most effective way to help improve the relationship between them" (p. 218).

If one or both partners could benefit from their own personal individual therapy, I refer them. This might be merited especially if character disorders or something requiring more intensive treatment is present. I almost always refer both partners even if I think that one could use it more than the other. I do it this way to preserve the integrity of the system – that each partner is contributing, in some way, to the relationship difficulty. Therefore, it is not unusual for each partner to have their own therapist while simultaneously doing couples work.

In working with commitment, it is best to give each partner the privacy to express their thoughts and feelings without fear of immediate reprisal by their mate. This is necessary because the kinds of questions asked that are needed to uncover a conflict can be sensitive, even painful. For example, sometimes one partner is not committed to the relationship because he/she is not physically attracted to the other or if one mate wants out but fears telling the other.

## Secrets

Many couples therapists ask what to do when one partner tells them a secret their counterpart is unaware of. Some of my colleagues believe that it should be agreed upon at the beginning of treatment that there will be no secrets held or protected by any partners or the therapist. I find this stance to hinder the art of the psychotherapeutic process. For example, if the therapist must reveal everything exposed, this will most likely enable partners to hide anything they deem especially controversial. In this situation neither couple nor the therapist will know if a durable commitment has a chance of being developed. Consider the following case.

Jim and his wife, Madelyn, sought couples therapy because Jim was having trouble achieving an erection, but he functioned fine with a woman he was having an affair with – a fact that especially hurt Madelyn. Although Jim would get an erection during foreplay, when it came to intercourse with Madelyn, his penis would become flaccid. Jim was cleared by his urologist of any organic problems and prescribed a drug for erectile dysfunction. He, however, procrastinated on filling his prescription, and when he did, he did not wait the required time it took to take effect, thereby sabotaging his erection. He did not need the medication when having sex with his affairee.

Couple sessions with Jim and Madelyn were going nowhere, and so I asked Jim to come in for an individual session. I was sure he was hiding something from me and Madelyn. It turned out that Jim had lost sexual desire for Madelyn because she had gained a lot of weight (i.e., approximately 200 pounds) since their marriage. Jim said that he still loved his wife but could no longer muster attraction for her. He was also angry about her weight gain.

My first recommendation was for Jim, an avid gym rat, to ask his wife if she would like to exercise with him. But he refused. He said it was her responsibility to lose weight and that she would slow him down if they worked out together. I then encouraged him to tell her the truth, but again he refused. Jim claimed you cannot talk to a woman about her weight. He said that it would cause too much pain and reprisal. He claimed he would rather leave Madelyn, which he was considering.

I did not find Madelyn to be a closed person, and she already suspected that Jim was hiding something. She even mentioned her weight gain as a potential problem, but Jim denied this in a conjoint session. Refusing to confront Madelyn enabled Jim to have his affair, which upset Madelyn even more. I could not reveal Jim's secret, but I eventually told the couple that they each merit individual therapy. Jim was already nearly "out the door." His commitment to his marriage was tenuous at best.

My refusal to reveal secrets can come with its consequences. Paula, a married female client, revealed to me in the initial contact that she had just ended a secretive affair to give her marriage a chance. She wanted to know if I would work with her and her husband, Wesley, under these conditions. She said that under no circumstances did she want to reveal her secret to Wesley because she was done with her affair and committed to working on her marriage. She said that if he was told about the affair, he would either never let go of it and use it to block the treatment or he would leave her. She claimed that Wesley did not forgive so easily and was obsessive compulsive. I told Paula that I would accept her terms and trust that the affair was indeed over.

The treatment had been going well for several months, and Paula decided it was safe to confess to Wesley about her affair. She said that since the marriage had gotten better, she did not think that her admission would do much damage. Paula did not consult me on this and in between sessions she revealed her secret. Not only did Wesley get mad at Paula, but he also took it out on me when it was revealed that I knew about the affair. This happened to me one other time in my career, and I was instantly fired. But I had a deep connection with Wesley, and although he was hurt, he accepted my excuse: that I could not reveal something told to me in confidence. The treatment took a month or two to get back on track, but it eventually did.

While my style of handling these kinds of secrets can backfire, I stand by my philosophy in pursuit of a more important objective: the survival of the relationship. If I cannot objectively treat a couple, I will reject them in the initial contact. This did happen on two occasions when married clients would ask me to help them with problems they were having with their affairees or lovers. Other therapists might not have a problem with this, but I feel that taking these kinds of cases may only feed into the pathology of all those involved.

## Refusing Treatment

There are those partners who refuse to attend therapy. Some of these individuals do so because: (1) they believe they can fix their issues without professional help (Barkley & Tartakovsky, 2023); (2) they fear being judged (Herzberg, 2023); (3) they see couples therapy as a punishment (Marie, 2021); or (4) they might believe it will make the relationship worse (Herzberg, 2023). Morin (2024) lists many reasons partners refuse to go to couples treatment; below are some that I have experienced most often:

- *Money* – They see therapy as too expensive and not worth the money.
- *Failure* – They believe therapy will not work.
- *Privacy* – They feel uncomfortable talking to a stranger about personal issues.
- *Embarrassment* – They feel embarrassed by having a problem.
- *Discomfort expressing feelings* – They feel too vulnerable expressing feelings.
- *Ganged up on* – They believe the therapist will side with their counterpart.

I would add from clinical experience that partners also refuse to go to couples therapy because they are avoidant, do not like responsibility, are angry at their partner, and because they believe that their counterpart is at fault and needs help more than they do. Some of these individuals may be too conflicted to work with, and so if I do decide to treat them, I make sure they know that I can only offer them what Kaplan (Personal communication, October 7, 1987) called "limited gains."

Working with one partner in need of couples therapy may help, but it is not preferable. Heitler (2022) found that working with one mate may damage a couple. I tend to agree, especially if the couple merit couples therapy. Individual therapists, if they have not had systemic training, may feel compelled to advocate for their clients, losing all sense of objectivity. I have spoken to therapists who, rather than assign responsibility to each partner, took the side of their client, thereby unbalancing the couple and exacerbating relational strife.

Most couples therapists may have to start with one partner but will try to move toward couples treatment. I make it a point to tell the partner that I will treat them for up to four sessions or until the absent partner agrees to come in, whichever comes first. If the absent partner decides to come after the allotted four sessions, I usually refer the couple to a different couples therapist. If the partner sees me anywhere from one to four individual sessions, I offer the absent partner the same number of individual sessions to maintain systemic integrity.

## Treatment Access

I also try and determine if the couple is geographically friendly. This is because couples who live a great distance from treatment are less likely to follow through with their commitment to therapy. Sometimes they simply misjudge the difficulty of their commute; other times it is an unconscious sabotage of the treatment. But I find it best to assess whether a couple is being realistic about their ability to attend sessions regularly. For example, when someone calls from another part of the state that requires a two- or more hour drive to see me, it is a good bet that they will be unable to commit the time it may need to help them.

Even those who insist on taking public transportation should be assessed. Are these people simply setting themselves and the therapist up for failure? Most people mean well, but they may not be aware of the sabotage their unconscious conflict with commitment has in store for them.

Randi called for an appointment but did not immediately let me know she was calling from another state. While she and her husband seemed like good candidates for couples therapy, their commute would have amounted to a total of six hours round trip, if traffic was cooperative. Although she was resistant, I was finally able to give her some referrals in her home state, where I once trained and had established some long-term professional relationships.

The distance a couple may need to travel for treatment, however, is no longer as significant a factor as it had been for many couples and couples therapists. Although there was a movement to treat people online in the mental health field before the pandemic, most therapists now use a hybrid model of treatment that consists of both going to their offices one or two days a week and treating the rest of their clients online. In fact, the 2021 COVID-19 Practitioner Survey conducted by the American Psychological Association (2021) found that 96% of all psychologists practice at least some online therapy and with little downside for therapist and client.

There are some differences in the online assessment process to determine a couple's commitment. It does seem easier for couples to avoid scheduling regular session times and to blame this on their work schedules, or interference from pets and family members who reside in the family home, where the couples are online. Some couples refuse or forget to lock the door of the room they are using, and animals and children routinely interrupt treatment. One couple allowed their maid to clean while they were in session, so I had to re-set limits out of concern for the couple's confidentiality. It was also profitable to process why the couple allowed this to begin with. Other couples claim that there are too many technical difficulties with online treatment to commit to regular therapy.

## Professional Expertise

Another way to help ensure commitment in couples therapy is for the therapist to assess whether he/she has the expertise to help the couple. There are many therapists who practice couples therapy with little to no training (Doherty, 2002). And there are couples therapists who are simply not skilled in treating certain areas such as sexual problems, domestic violence, or trauma.

If both the couple and the therapist collude in ignoring the competence of the therapist, it might be a forgone conclusion that the couple will eventually be dissatisfied with their treatment and prematurely terminate. The therapist too may become frustrated and begin to feel clinically impotent. To this point, I have known colleagues over the years who have decided to treat a problem they had little expertise in. Those who succeeded in seeking out appropriate supervision learned something new and helped their clients. Those who used clients as an experiment eventually became frustrated, as did their clients, and eventually had to refer the couple to someone more appropriate.

## First Session

In the first appointment, whether it is live or online, the couples therapist should keep the agreed-upon structure of the treatment intact (Doherty, 2002; Weeks & Fife, 2014). For example, reducing the fee without a solid therapeutic reason may only enable the couple's lack of commitment. Couples therapy is often argumentative and can escalate to violence quickly. Once a couple begin to fight about their commitment issues, the therapist may not be given many chances to intervene and restore order. The couples therapist must maintain control throughout the treatment process, so the therapy does not fall into chaos. I'll say more about this in Chapter 6.

In the first session, the couples therapist gets the chance to observe the couple's dynamic and whether they will abide by the structure of the therapy. I am always watching for signs that one or both partners are not committed to each other or the treatment process. Some partners will never admit they are not invested – these individuals might fear upsetting the committed partner. But their level of commitment will show in therapy.

The types and tendencies of each partner discussed in Chapter 2 will be on full display. The committed partner may enter the first session pursuing attachment, love, passion, or greater intimacy from their partner. This individual may demonstrate a need to please or appear anxious, dependent, or needy. They may suffer from low self-worth or exhibit masochistic tendencies. The uncommitted partner may be distancing from their partner and complain about feeling suffocated or smothered by their counterpart's need for intimacy and passion. They may be distrusting, have a survivalist mentality, or present as greedy or narcissistic. The therapist should be aware of both individual tendencies and systemic dynamics.

There may be hints of the couple's conflict with commitment in the first session. I always tell trainees and supervisees: "If something makes you scratch their head, you should follow it because it may lead to the conflict." But you cannot be certain of the conflict until a full assessment is completed, including an examination of each partner's family of origin and life experience.

The formal assessment phase usually takes one to two sessions depending on the complexity of the case, but the therapist continues to assess throughout treatment. I usually begin the family of origin examination in the first session by drawing two genograms in my notes, one for each partner. I then begin by asking each partner, in turn, a series of questions. I take my time and do not move to the next partner until I have gotten the material I need to make a proper assessment. This may take an entire session and feel unbalanced. But I let the couple know that the next session will be dedicated to the other partner. I also believe this style enables each partner to listen to the other's story and increases the chances of developing mutual empathy.

Many therapists have a different style of approach. Those with behavioral leanings are typically not interested in taking a history and instead focus on helping the client change their present behavior. Others focus on the present systemic dynamics of the couple. Because I am presenting an integrative conflict model made up of psychoanalytic conflict theory and psychodynamic family of origin work, I believe that taking a couple's history is the most efficient way to assess a relationship with accuracy.

I do not mean to suggest that after the genograms are complete, the assessment is over. The genogram and interactional data only give the therapist a framework from which to draw. Couples will continue throughout the treatment process to add or change information. The following section will give an indication of the kinds of questions asked by the therapist.

## Questions for the Genogram

There are several questions I pose to each partner during the first session or two that, if answered honestly, can provide the couples therapist with significant clinical information about the couple, especially in the context of commitment. For example, the interview should tell the therapist which of the key ingredients in commitment the couple are having difficulty: attachment, love, intimacy, or passion. Although this is most likely evident in the couple's interaction, it should confirm which partner plays the role of the committed and which plays the role of the uncommitted. And most importantly, it can lead the therapist to a couple's shared conflict with commitment.

The questions range from basic to more complex and may be questions about a partner's past or present. In sum, the questions are aimed at: (1) identifying which role each partner plays in their couple interaction (i.e., the committed or uncommitted partner); (2) recognizing the specific symptoms the couple display in the context of commitment such as difficulties with love, attachment, intimacy and passion (including sex); and (3) uncovering the shared conflict with romantic commitment that may be behind the couple's symptoms and their lack of durability.

Questions asked of each partner and their answers are recorded on each partner's respective genogram. When it is not their turn to be interviewed, the other partner is required to sit quietly in attendance and listen to their counterpart's story. Many of these individuals have told me that in doing so they have learned things about their partner that they never knew.

Partners are allowed to disrupt a response if they deem it incorrect or if they can add something significant to the conversation, but they are not allowed to take the session over when it is their partner's turn to be questioned. Most of the questions are asked with both partners in the room, but there are some that merit more confidentiality and are asked in individual sessions. These might include more personal or sensitive questions related to attraction, infidelity, or sexual abuse, to name a few. Questions marked by an asterisk signify those questions that the therapist should consider only asking in an individual session.

There is no one question that can expose a conflict with commitment, and the therapist should not solely rely on the couple's interactional dynamic for a full complete explanation of their commitment conflict. It is the accumulation of data from their interactions and the many different questions and answers that can help a couples therapist to uncover a conflict with commitment and determine how the conflict is related to any of the symptoms a couple is experiencing. The reader can find an exhaustive list of general questions for the genogram by consulting past writings (Betchen, 2022; Betchen & Davidson, 2018). The following are questions that I believe will lead to uncovering a conflict specifically with commitment. The relevance of each question is supported by appropriate research data when possible.

### How do you identify ethnically, racially, and religiously?

Most older couples laugh when I ask this question. They see it as a reflection of the current generation. But sociocultural variables matter when it comes to assessing romantic commitment. For example, couples who come from countries that arrange marriages are more likely to feel obligated to commit to their relationship. Pressure from family and friends helps a couple to honor the arrangement even if they no longer live in their country of origin. Also, most of these individuals are virgins when they meet and, in my clinical experience, did not get a chance to determine if they are sexually compatible. In this context, many discover there is a problem after they are married.

Being in love in an arranged marriage is also not as important as loving and honoring one another and one's family and community. Arranged marriage is not the same as a forced marriage; however, it is still a collective, transactional dynamic, not necessarily a loving, passionate, intimate union based on one's individual needs and desires (Tahir, 2021). Making a commitment under these conditions, especially in a country that stresses individualism like the United States, makes a conflict for these couples far more probable. According to the World Population Review (2024), the following countries still arrange marriage: India, Iran, Iraq, China, Japan, Indonesia, and South Korea. Bangladesh and Pakistan have forced marriages.

Race can also be a factor in romantic commitment. Kogan et al. (2016) found that harsh, unsupportive parenting and racial discrimination contribute to commitment-related behavior in Black men. This finding is in tune with my clinical experience working with Black couples. Girlfriends complained about an almost phobic response to marriage from their male counterparts, and wives complained about infidelity or a lack of commitment to family life. Many of these women scolded their male partners as if they were irresponsible adolescents – something the men predictably responded angrily to. In their research, Abrams et al. (2018) found that Black women viewed Black men as having difficulty connecting and committing to their partners and families. But they were empathic and believed social barriers were to blame.

Religion has its rules, and many couples I have seen put it before their personal feelings and desires. A female client married a man because he was a fellow Christian sanctioned by her family and community. She thought she was doing the right thing at the time but never considered that she was not physically attracted to him. For this woman, the relationship was transactional – she was committed because she was a rule follower, not because the relationship contained the ingredients of commitment such as love, passion, and intimacy. While this may be a dramatic example of the power religion can have on commitment, I have treated numerous Catholics over the years who claimed that divorce is not an option. They, in fact, feel that they cannot break a pledge they made to their partner and to God.

Religion, however, can also have a more positive binding impact on relationships and for good reason. According to Call and Heaton (1997), couples who believe in religion make stronger marital commitments. Sullivan (2001) found that religious married couples have happier, more stable relationships.

Some studies have found that couples who share the same faith are more durable than others (Aman et al., 2021). Research from the Pew Research Center's Religious Landscape Survey (2015) found that approximately two thirds (64%) of those surveyed reported that it was important to be married to someone of the same faith to have a successful marriage. Only 24% believed that being married to someone of a different faith had the same impact, and 17% felt this way when only one partner was religiously affiliated. Collisson (2022) found that interfaith relationships can create more stress and limit social and emotional connectedness. I have found that religious difference can be used by a couple to engage in control struggles (Betchen, 2022).

### How do you identify sexually?

I rarely ask this question because it is often easy to identify a couple's sexual identity when I meet them. But I do think it is important, especially for the straight therapist to better understand the dynamics of same-sex couples. Even though same-sex couples have long suffered from the stigma that they are unable to commit to a long-term relationship, studies have found that they in fact experience similar levels of commitment and intimacy as do other population groups (Joyner et al., 2019).

There are also many similarities between commitment in same-sex and straight couples with the exception that male gay couples show more of a preference for nonmonogamy (Rostosky et al., 2006). According to the Gay Male Center, approximately 50% of gay male couples practice some form of nonmonogamy (Blum, 2024). This may take many forms: (1) a polyamorous relationship or loving relationships with others; (2) a closed relationship with others; (3) an open relationship in which the couple retains emotional intimacy within the primary relationship while pursuing additional sexual partners; and (4) a swinging relationship in which partners pursue other couples for sex (Levine et al., 2018).

I have seen a small but increasing number of nonmonogamous couples or couples who practiced consensual nonmonogamy (CNM) over the past several years as the popularity of this relationship style has increased (Gupta et al., 2023). Moors et al. (2021) reported that approximately one in nine people engaged in polyamory – a form of CNM – and according to a large U.S. survey, 4% of the respondents who were partnered practiced CNM (Levine et al., 2018).

While it may seem easy to exclude nonmonogamous couples from a discussion on romantic commitment, others would argue that one can be both committed and practice CNM simultaneously (Kelberga & Martinsone, 2021). Many CNM individuals are married or cohabitating, have multiple long-term relationships, and are invested in the success of their relationships. Therefore, a couple's sexual preference should not be automatically perceived by the therapist as a lack of commitment to the primary relationship. The concept of commitment is equally important to both same-sex and straight couples, but some differences do exist as well as ever present institutional discrimination. The couples therapist must be careful not to assess same-sex couples from a strict heteronormative model. This will only exacerbate any pre-existing stigmas that many CNM couples already face in their families and the larger community. Research has indicated that too many therapists discourage CNM and risk premature termination (Schechinger et al., 2018).

Asking about a couple's sexual preferences and how they handle them may reveal something about their level of commitment. For example, while many CNM couples do fine, many break the rules they established and experience severe relationship difficulty; CNM or any form of open relationship can be a slippery slope (Betchen, 2013).

### Are you married, cohabitating, or dating, and for how long?

According to data from the U.S. Census Bureau, more adults find cohabitation an acceptable arrangement (Horowitz et al., 2019). But the couples therapist should still consider marriage to be a helpful predictor of the ability to commit in a relationship in part, because of its link to tradition and its emotional and legal binding. The Institute for Family Studies found that married individuals rate higher in commitment than those living together (Wilcox et al., 2019). Stanley and Rhoades (2023) reported that those who lived together before marriage had a greater chance of divorcing. And a study in *Demographic Research* found that 54% of first-time cohabitators experienced the breakup of their relationship within six years (Mernitz, 2018).

Many people think that living together and marrying are one in the same. I, however, think the difference is significant. Living together, metaphorically speaking, leaves an escape hatch for either partner to bolt from the relationship. Marriage brings with it all the emotional, financial, and legal problems that make it much more difficult and costly to escape. People with relationship commitment issues are more comfortable cohabitating.

The length of a relationship is also an important variable in this discussion and should be considered on a continuum. For example, a couple who has been dating exclusively for several years is more indicative of an ability to commit. A couple who has been living together for an equal amount of time may indicate even more commitment but not as much as a long-term married couple. The point being is the therapist should gather as much detail about the time length and quality of the relationships to determine the durability of commitment.

People who have an ability to attach and commit are less likely to have a conflict with committing and more likely to have longer-term relationships. But I also happen to believe that partners who have been together exclusively for their entire lives may have little confidence in their ability to attract others or a fear of separation. Some of these couples may even appear enmeshed or symbiotic. Individuals such as these may also have a conflict with commitment represented by their enmeshment or symbiosis.

The average length of a partner's "past" relationships might also be of some value. For example, an individual may have a pattern of ending a relationship after five years. It is as if this person has an internal timer that reminds him/her that their commitment quota has been met. I refer to this mechanism as an "internal egg timer," based on the kind of timer my mother used when boiling eggs. When the timer went off, the eggs were sufficiently boiled. In the context of romantic relationships, when the individual's timer goes off, he/she feels compelled to end the relationship.

*How long did you date before you married, moved in, or decided to date exclusively?*

I believe the answer to this question is especially useful when assessing a conflict with romantic commitment. Francis-Tan and Mialon (2015) found that dating your potential spouse at least three years before marrying them significantly reduced the chances of divorce. I believe that a long dating history, especially if it is exclusive, may be a sign of an ability to commit. But those individuals who put off living together or marrying for an inordinate amount of time may reflect a conflict with commitment.

Some couples marry soon after meeting. This choice may be impulsive and therefore merits attention to see if it reflects a conflict with commitment. Zach and his girlfriend of two months, Nellie, presented for treatment because Nellie was seriously threatening to end the relationship. She also made it clear she was not going to commit to treatment. Zach said that he was especially confused because Nellie was the initiator of the relationship and that she relentlessly pursued him. He even claimed that Nellie literally tore his clothes off on their first date and within four dates she brought up the idea of marriage. Nellie seemed just as confused about her need to leave Zach, but she was sure that she had to go. Nellie had a track record of these impulsive behaviors, which start off intense but quickly wane.

*Where and how did you meet?*

Rosenfeld et al. (2019) found that online dating is now the most popular way to meet people. They reported that it has replaced "meeting through friends." And that it can work for those wanting a long-term commitment. Vogels and McClain (2023) found: "one-in-ten partnered adults – meaning those who are married, living with a partner or in a committed relationship – met their current significant other through a dating site or app" (p. 1). A large-scale Forbes Health Survey found that approximately 70% of people who met on a dating app led to an exclusive relationship (Booth, 2024).

Nevertheless, people with significant commitment problems tend to choose places to meet that will challenge the odds of fulfilling a commitment. For example, some couples meet on certain dating sites or apps that are better known for "hooking-up" and contain their fair share of sex addicts or sexually compulsive individuals, adulterous people, professional sex workers, or scammers. Long-term commitment is not necessarily the objective of many of these individuals.

*How many sexual relationships did you have before you met your partner?\**

Wolfinger (2018) found that partners who have had sex with fewer people were happier in marriage. Stewart-Williams et al. (2017) discovered that initially, the number of partners a person had sex with did not determine whether someone would date them. But as the number of partners increased, so did the reluctance of both men and women to enter a relationship with these individuals. Reasons varied, but people viewed those who had many sex partners as promiscuous and less likely to commit. A high number of sexual partners may be indicative of a conflict with commitment, so this question is worth asking.

### Does your current relationship remind you of any past relationships?

I always take a relationship history in part because people tend to replicate or re-experience commitment issues time and again (Martin, 2018). For example, Ray had little to no sexual interest in his wife. In taking his relationship history, however, I discovered that he had also developed low sexual desire, which was the cause of divorce from his first wife and many significant girlfriends from his past.

Another example is that of Terri, who claimed to have slept with over 100 men. When she married, she admittedly could not commit to one person and asked her husband to open the marriage. One rule I have is "If a partner is unusually inexperienced or too experienced, a conflict with commitment may be operating."

### Were you ever engaged or married before, and for how long?

Prior marriage, if it was reasonably healthy and long-lasting, may be an indication of an individual's ability to attach and commit. However, assuming the ability to commit with someone who has been engaged without more information may prove precipitous. It is not so unusual to find people with commitment conflicts engaged numerous times. These individuals seem to find a way out of the relationship before it culminates in marriage. According to Rodman (2018), a problem with taking the next step in a relationship could be a sign of difficulty with commitment.

### Who ended your past relationships, and why?

The answer to this question will tell if the partner has a history of getting out of relationships. It is especially telling if the reasons for the breakups seem frivolous or manufactured, only serving to allow an individual to escape commitment. Alice always found something wrong with her dates. One man was too short, another was too poor, and another dressed inappropriately. When she wanted to leave the relationship, she called upon whatever dislike she had discovered and escalated its significance until she convinced herself to end the relationship. Once she accomplished this, she felt justified in her decision.

### Do you have a history of recycling relationships?

Some people "breakup and makeup" repeatedly with the same partner. This is referred to as *relationship cycling* (Dailey et al., 2009). According to Vennum et al. (2014), people who repeatedly cycle "are at greater risk for further cycling and experiencing greater constraints to permanently ending the relationship, greater uncertainty in their relationship's future, and lower satisfaction" (p. 410).

Maintaining what she referred to as her "Catholic values," Brenda wanted to remain a virgin until marriage, but Michael did not want to wait. Blaming Brenda, he would break up with her to date and sleep with other women but would soon return to her. Brenda tolerated Michael's behavior because she empathized with his position. But she also thought that once the couple married, Michael would no longer need to stray. Michael, however, was used to his lifestyle and continued to have short-lived flings after marriage until Brenda finally threatened to leave him. He then agreed to stop their relationship recycling dynamic.

### How is your sex life, and is there sufficient passion?*

Passion, in of itself cannot hold a relationship together. According to Ben-Zeév (2019), without friendship a relationship cannot endure long term. Nevertheless, having a healthy desire for your partner can only add to relationship commitment. The therapist should inquire as to whether the partner feels there is passion in the relationship. This is important to know, especially if a couple has a sexual problem. Many of these couples have little to no foreplay in their sex lives signaling a passionless relationship. Some couples in treatment have called their passionless relationships, "robotic."

### Have you had any problems with sex in your past relationships?

The answer to this question can tell the therapist whether there is a "pattern" of sexual distress or failure in the partner's past romantic relationships. This information might, in turn, point to a conflict with commitment exhibited by the couple's sex dysfunction. For example, if a man has a history of delayed ejaculation, he may also have a pattern of withholding affection.

### Have you ever cheated on your current or past partners?*

Again, the answer to this question should give you an idea as to the level of commitment the partner is capable of. According to Gunther (2011), approximately 50% of committed partners stay faithful. Selterman et al. (2019) found low commitment to a relationship is one of the major causes of cheating. Most chronic cheaters are in the throes of an underlying conflict with commitment.

### Were there any addictions in your family?

According to a survey conducted and released in 2022 by the U.S. Department of Health and Human Services (2023) through the Substance Abuse and Mental Health Services Administration, 48.7 million people aged 12 or older have a substance abuse disorder with drug or alcohol. According to Bergman (2024), up to 20 million people have a gambling problem. And according to the Mayo Clinic, up to 24 million sex addicts are in the Unites States (Gleeson, 2022). It should be noted that some scholars have called into question the term *sex addiction*, preferring to use "out-of-control sexual behavior" (Braun-Harvey & Vigorito, 2015). These individuals believe that the label *sex addiction* is not supported by adequate research and is pejorative.

Addicts have commitment issues in romantic relationships because most can only commit to their addiction of choice. This means that partners of addicts always take seconds to the addiction itself and are often used as an object to help the addict to feed or maintain the addiction. Addicts get drunk or stoned or are busy gambling away the family savings. They often forget their partner's birthdays or their children's recitals and plays. Many lie and steal only to support their habit.

Simply put, addicts cannot be fully committed to a romantic relationship while in the throes of an addiction. They cannot "love" (Collins, 2023). This is in part why some partners of addicts join them in the addiction – to stay close to them. This way they have some semblance of a connection.

### Do you use porn, and if so, how often?

According to the National Couples and Pornography Survey 2021, 90% of the couples who reported no porn use in their relationship had the highest levels of relationship stability and commitment (Wheatley Institute, 2021). But some researchers have found that porn use can enhance relationship quality. For example, Kohut et al. (2021) found that porn can be good for a relationship if partners agree on the type of porn and enjoy sharing it. Hakkim et al. (2022) found that porn use in relationships can improve sexual arousal, lead to more orgasms, increase sexual interest, and enable sexual experimentation. However, there is a difference between porn use and compulsive porn use. Weiss (2020) claimed that compulsive porn users always find themselves leading stressful, compartmentalized lives. Little intimacy is involved as the objectified partner takes second place to the porn use.

Excessive use of porn is indeed one way to distance from a partner. But the therapist will need to be detailed in asking this question because the partner could be getting plenty of sex from their counterpart but not the specific sexual need they crave. If, for example, the partner who is captivated by porn has a particular "delicacy" that their counterpart is not satisfying, there is a good chance the relationship is lacking in passion, intimacy, and, in turn, commitment.

### What role did you play in your family of origin?

What role an individual played in the family or origin may tell the therapist something about their ability to commit. For example, if a client was parentified as a child, or if they were burdened with the primary caregiver job at an inappropriately young age, it is possible that as an adult he/she may be torn between obligation and freedom. Taking on more responsibility such as a serious relationship might trigger a feeling of being reparentified or re-burdened.

**Do you have any siblings, and if so, are they in relationships?**

While some researchers incorporate the importance of multiple sibling influences in their study of family dynamics (McHale et al., 2012), I tend not to ask too many questions about siblings. But I am interested in families in which every sibling is experiencing similar relationship symptoms to determine if they share a conflict with commitment. Especially telling of a potential conflict with commitment is a family in which all or almost all siblings have been divorced, and some more than once.

**Where you ever abused in any way, as a child or as an adult?***

People who were abused or neglected as a child will most likely have difficulty trusting in romantic relationships. And if the abuse was by the hand of someone whom they considered safe, such as a parent, allowing someone to get close and trusting them as an adult will be even more difficult.

Herrero et al. (2018) found that in adulthood, children of abuse are more likely to choose abusive partners. The Office for National Statistics (2017) reported that more than half (51%) of abused children will be domestically abused as adults. And female victims of child abuse are more likely to choose abusive men for adult relationships (Herrero et al., 2018). Related to this dynamic is "the cycle of abuse," a four-stage pattern consisting of tension, incident, reconciliation, and calm, which continuously repeats itself (Gillette, 2022).

To help determine whether a conflict with commitment is at play in the context of abuse, I look for two indicators: (1) abused individual replicates the abuse by repeatedly choosing abusive partners and (2) abused individual has difficulty ending abusive relationships.

**Did your parents quarrel, and if so, what did they usually fight about?**

The answer to this question may reveal that the partner's parents fought about any one of the ingredients that make up commitment. Did they fight because one or both did not feel loved? Did they fight because there was little to no passion in their relationship? Did they complain about a lack of intimacy? Children who grew up with quarreling parents are less likely to form healthy attachments in romantic relationships (Mandriota, 2021).

**Are your parents still married?**

The answer to this question may tell the therapist if the partner's parents served as role models of commitment. Research has indicated that those whose parents never married, or who have divorced, reported lowest relationship quality in terms of commitment, among other variables (Rhoades et al., 2012).

**Did your parents separate repeatedly?**

Some parents separate numerous times, and even though they might not divorce, research has found that this can cause posttraumatic stress and attachment problems in children (Briggs-Gowan et al., 2019). Couples who are on and off send a mixed message to their children: you cannot live with a partner comfortably, and you cannot live without one. It will then not be unusual to see the child replicate this dynamic in their adult romantic relationships.

### Did either parent ever threaten to leave?

Even if a parent does not physically leave home, the threat of it can lead to feelings of insecurity and a fear of instability that may make it hard for the individual to commit as an adult. Ever since Kathleen could remember, her mother threatened to leave her father. As an adult Kathleen feared abandonment and made sure that she left before any of her partners did.

### To the best of your knowledge, did either parent ever have an affair?

Research has indicated that people whose parents cheated are more likely to cheat in their adult relationships (Negash & Morgan, 2016). I have seen men who have followed their cheating fathers because cheating on a partner fit their definition of what a "real man" does.

### How long have you been at your present place of employment?

Sometimes a partner's record of low commitment in other contexts can tell the therapist whether the individual can commit in a relationship. I have always found that broadening the context for couples allows them to see the pervasiveness of a conflict (Betchen, 2022, 2024; Betchen & Davidson, 2018).

### Do you usually keep your promises?

According to Kanngiesser et al. (2023), promises are like voluntary commitments. And people who keep their promises to partners demonstrate a commitment to themselves and the relationship. On the contrary, people who consistently break their word are more likely to have commitment problems in their romantic relationships.

### Do you start to feel uncomfortable the closer you seem to get to someone?

People with a commitment conflict will feel uncomfortable the closer they get to committing. I have seen this dynamic in romantic relationships, but it can also interfere with achieving other aspirations. According to Brogaard (2015), falling in love with someone who is commitment-phobic may be a nightmare. The author contends these people can get close to things, but they fear getting close to people. Jacobsen (2023) reports that people with commitment phobia become very anxious the closer they get in a romantic relationship. Most will ask for "space."

### Have either parent ever told you to never give up on or quit something?

Some parents give their children the message to never quit or give up. These individuals may internalize this message and stick with something to the finish. While this can be a positive message, if the situation is abusive, that same child may not be able to extricate themselves from a bad situation. That is, sometimes quitting something is a good thing. It can save the individual a lot of pain and time.

*Do you and your partner talk, especially about personal issues?*

This can tell the therapist if there is a sufficient connection and if the couple can be intimate. As mentioned, intimacy is a key ingredient in a romantic relationship and a problem with it could signify a conflict with commitment. According to Khalifian and Barry (2020), sharing is a way to build trust and intimacy with another.

*Do you and your partner share interests?*

Sharing interests can be correlated with romantic commitment. A couple that enjoys the same hobbies and passions in life may commit more easily to each other. According to Betchen (2020), couples that share interests have healthier, more durable relationships.

*Do you trust your partner?*

Relationships void of trust are usually void of intimacy. There will never be a sense of safety and security. According to George (2024), partners who betray their counterparts are resistant to commitment.

*Do you and your partner love each other, or are you both in love with each other?**

Love is reciprocal in healthy relationships (Applebury, 2020). It is also the glue to commitment. Love can indeed hold a couple together but, as noted, being "in love" makes people want to be together. One can love a pet, but being in love is a strong indicator of romantic commitment. You may feel as if there is no one else in the world who would suit you better. There is very little that is transactional about this kind of relationship. Much of it may, in fact, be unconditional.

## Clinical Case Assessments

### Assessing Sean and Jessica (See Figure 5.2)

Sean and Jessica had been married for 15 years. Sean was a 40-year-old contractor and Jessica was a 36-year-old secretary at an insurance company. The couple had two young children.

#### Initial Contact

Sean called to request couples' sessions and said his wife Jessica was in favor of it. The couple have known each other since the eighth grade. They lived in the same development and attended the same elementary school.

Sean claimed that he loved Jessica and always has, but in the past two years, she has been distant. He mentioned her low sex drive, but he was alluding to something much broader. I asked if he could identify an incident that might have triggered Jessica's change in behavior, but he could not identify any. He claimed that her distancing was a gradual process.

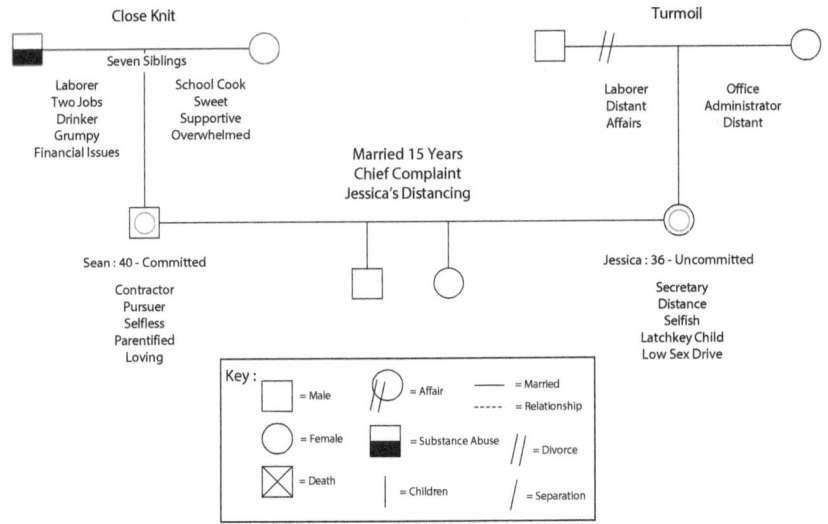

*Figure 5.2* Sean and Jessica.

He said that he and Jessica seemed inseparable for many years and that they routinely had sex every weekend up until about two years ago. I then asked Sean if Jessica gave him a reason for her behavior, and he said that she was just as confused as he was and that both would like answers. I suspected much more was going on with this relationship, but I gave the couple a first appointment after going over the treatment structure with him.

*First Session*

The first session validated the feeling I got from the initial contact: that Sean played the role of the committed partner and Jessica played the uncommitted partner. Sean, a ruggedly handsome man, was very much in love with Jessica. He was saddened and confused with her indifferent behavior toward him and especially her seemingly absent sex drive and lack of passion. He said that there was a time when he and Jessica could talk about anything, but he feels she has shut him out. He also astutely stated that she does not seem to need him anymore. He mentioned that although he did not have much experience by comparison, he did not think that Jessica ever had a high sex drive, but he saw her as beautiful, and sexy, nonetheless. He also liked her personality, and they seemed to have shared interests. Jessica made it a point that she loved the fact that Sean had a big, close-knit, fun-loving family. Apparently, Sean's parents routinely had big parties and had always made Jessica feel welcome.

Sean appeared quiet and humble. He spoke in a soft voice, which belied his muscular physique. Neither he nor Jessica was college educated but both worked, and Sean was a good provider. Sean made it clear that his treatment goal was to find out what Jessica needed from him to return to the wife she once was. He was a pleaser and willing to do anything for Jessica. Jessica was not as clear about her objectives. She, in fact, seemed vague and somewhat confused about her lack of interest in Sean and their relationship. She did say that she would love to better understand what was happening to her. She added, "Any women would love to have Sean. He is handsome, kind, and considerate. I am just not interested in the relationship the way I used to be."

### Genogram

Sean was raised the oldest of eight siblings in a close-knit Irish Catholic family. His siblings all lived relatively close to one another and socialized frequently. Sean loved his siblings but at times did feel burdened by them. Apparently, Sean's father held two jobs and his mother served as a school cook, so Sean had to look after his siblings and keep the house in order. Sean was by all accounts parentified with a history of caretaking. One girlfriend from his past was raised in a broken, dysfunctional home. Sean took her into his family and admittedly rescued her.

Sean described his father as a distant, "grumpy" man who was overwhelmed having to support such a big family. He sometimes drank heavily but was not abusive. If anything, Sean said that his father usually fell asleep when he had too much to drink. Alcohol notwithstanding, Sean's father worked long, hard hours and was unable to spend much time with his children. Sean described his mother as sweet, supportive, as well as overwhelmed.

Sean claimed that despite some financial difficulties, the family threw big parties, and all members were supportive of one another. He did wonder, however, whether these parties served to distract the family from their difficulties. Sean claimed that feelings were never really discussed in the family and that everyone had a job to do to survive. He especially did not want to further burden his parents with any complaints. He said that his parents got along reasonably well, especially when his father was sober. He joked that they probably worked too much to fight. He did, however, see both as tired and felt bad for them.

Sean was not a drinker, and he claimed that he had never experienced any type of abuse. He was not on any medication, although he did appear somewhat depressed given his present situation. He reported no fetishes and described himself as sexually conservative. "I am a one-woman man," he said. He claimed that he had no need for porn and that he had always been faithful to Jessica.

Jessica was an only child. Her parents fought most of her life, mostly about money and her father's affairs. They divorced when Jessica was about to start high school. As children, Jessica and Sean had a mutual group of friends, and as they progressed through school, they became closer. By the time they were juniors in high school, they were inseparable. Sean said that he always knew he was going to marry Jessica. They went to both junior and senior proms together and were a popular couple in high school.

Jessica described her father as a laborer who was never home. She said that he always seemed to have a girlfriend who he preferred to spend time and money on, and he rarely spent any time with her. Although her mother was more accessible, she worked as an office administrator and had little time for Jessica. Jessica considered herself a "latchkey child." Even with her attractiveness and robust social life, Jessica said that most of the time she was lost and lonely.

Sean and Jessica got married as soon as they both graduated from high school. Sean was very happy to have Jessica as his wife. He said he could not see being with anyone else. Jessica was less sure of herself and her motivations. She said that she had always loved Sean but sometimes wondered if he was the right guy for her. She questioned whether she loved his family and the close-knit connections more than she loved him. When I distinguished the difference between loving and being in love, she said that was not in love with Sean but that she did love him and felt terrible for the way she was treating him. "All he ever did was take care of me and this is how I repay him."

Because I did not want to risk exposing something detrimental to the relationship too soon, I requested an individual session with each partner following the first conjoint session. As suspected, Sean was bewildered by his wife's behavior, but he did tell me that the couple's sex life was never "great." He said that he was always under the impression that Jessica could live without sex. He stated that he would like nothing better than to see her happy and aroused by him, but overall, he was satisfied with her. She certainly was not a hassle to be with and allowed him to do what he wanted in and outside the relationship. She was also very easy to get along with and his family loved her.

The individual session with Jessica was different. Jessica again reiterated how handsome Sean was but said that she had no physical attraction for him. She said that she loved him, but it was more like a lifelong friendship. Jessica claimed that she did, in fact, have a strong libido but for others, not Sean. She also said that she was considering divorce but feared losing Sean's friendship and family. She also feared she would be racked with guilt if she left him.

### Assessment Summary

Jessica was always in conflict about her commitment to Sean, but she was only vaguely conscious of it. When she was young, she saw Sean as a handsome, popular guy. She was not aware of her neediness and that she was more attracted to his large close-knit family – the family she never had. But she did sense a void. This explains some of Jessica's flirting with other men, temptation to have affairs, and eventually her low sexual desire and distancing – they were all symptoms of a conflict with commitment.

Jessica's conflict: She wanted to be taken care of by Sean. She loved being a member of his large family and appreciated him as a best friend. But she also longed for real romantic love, sexual passion, and intimacy. In sum, Jessica was tired of the trade she made between being taken care of by Sean versus relying on herself and taking the risk to find someone than better fit her needs. Without reconciling this conflict, she would have difficulty committing to Sean.

As noted, Jessica played the role of the uncommitted partner, and she appeared as a somewhat selfish distancer in the relationship dynamic. Her genogram indicated that she was a lonely child from a broken home. Her distant father and mother provided her with little nurturing, and her parents' divorce only exacerbated her neediness and loneliness. She unconsciously chose Sean to survive rather than because she was in love with him. This helps to explain her strong attachment to his family.

Because of Sean's internalized parentification, he had difficulty considering his own needs beyond that of caring for others. He unconsciously chose Jessica to rescue and treated her like a child for most of their relationship and subsequent marriage. He even called her his "wounded bird." Even in sex he focused on her needs.

Sean played the role of the committed, selfless partner. He was a pleaser and asked for very little in return. He was also the pursuer to Jessica's distancer. The relationship between the two was also somewhat transactional, and if Jessica was unhappy, he took it personally and it became a project that he needed to fix.

Sean's conflict: He needed to rescue Jessica to replicate in his familiar parentified role. Although burdened with responsibility, it's the only role he knew how to behave in a relationship. But he also wanted a committed woman who would meet his needs. Jessica was not fully developed enough to meet anyone's emotional needs, and the fact that he chose her predominantly for the purpose of nurturing all but guaranteed that he, too, had a conflict with commitment.

### Clinical Recommendations

To balance this couple's shared conflict with commitment and achieve a durable relationship, each partner must come to recognize the role their families of origin have played in helping to create this conflict. Jessica already knew that she was not committed to her marriage – she was never truly committed to her relationship with Sean. And she was never attracted to him as a lover. She must therefore either accept her marriage for its limitations and fix what is fixable, especially in the contexts of love, sex, and passion, or let Sean and his family go. Letting go of Sean's family might bring on significant anxiety and depression, but Jessica cannot have it both ways. Adult women make adult decisions. Jessica must continue to mature and take care of herself rather than look to others to meet her needs.

Sean must own his parentification and his need to rescue. He must come to realize that he is worthy of getting his needs met beyond caretaking and pleasing others. If he can, he may be better able to cope with the loss of Jessica. He may also become more gravitated to competent, adult women who could meet his needs. To do so, however, he will have to suffer the loss of the specialness that parentification brings. When a parentified person loses a needy partner, it is a loss of self-esteem and self-worth, but this sacrifice might increase the couple's durability.

### Assessing Lee and Jenna (See Figure 5.3)

Lee and Jenna were a couple in their late 30s. Lee was in finance, and Jenna split her duties between running her own business and being housewife and mother. The couple had been married for 15 years. They had two young children.

#### Initial Contact

Lee made the initial call. He said that he had yet to tell his wife, but he was not sure he wanted to stay married to her. He was attracted to another

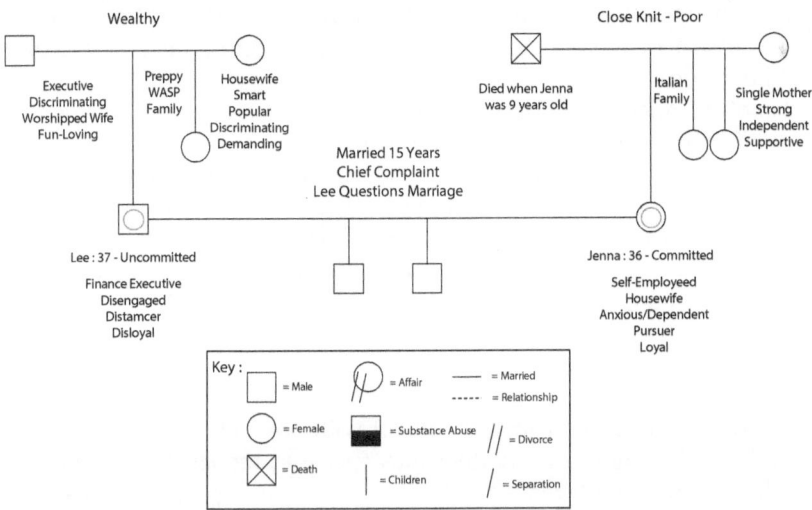

Figure 5.3 Lee and Jenna.

woman whom he perceived to be "more his type." He added that he and his wife, Jenna, are very different and that he never should have married her. Lee's parents agreed with him – they thought, "He could have done better." When I asked why he did marry Jenna, Lee sheepishly said that he did not want to break her heart.

It was clear that Lee was always conflicted about committing to Jenna even though he seemed to like her as a person. He felt that Jenna loved him far more than he loved her. He said that Jenna is looking forward to treatment. She complains that he is quick-tempered and hypercritical of her. Lee said he was nervous about therapy and would not have called me if Jenna did not push him.

### First Session

The first thing I noticed was the difference in looks. Lee was a tall, preppy man and Jenna was a short, dark, Italian woman. But the couple shared a lot of interests and hobbies. For example, both were golfers and skiers and enjoyed the company of their children. It was also evident, however, that Jenna was very angry and disappointed with Lee. She claimed to love Lee but felt that although he was an engaged father, he was a disengaged husband, especially over the last two years. She said that he only initiates sex when he is "really horny" and that it feels robotic or lacking in passion. Jenna said that Lee focuses on his own needs, and as soon as he has achieved orgasm, he jumps out of bed. She claimed there is no longer any affection in the marriage, and even when she initiates it, she receives little in return. She felt there was never much passion in her marriage, and there is less now than ever.

Lee sat quietly; he neither confirmed nor disconfirmed Jenna's accusations. He was disengaged. I wondered whether he was waiting for the perfect moment to tell Jenna that he wanted out of the marriage. But I also knew from speaking with him on the telephone that he did not want to hurt her. Lee saw Jenna as a great mother and was reluctant to upset the children with a separation or divorce. But it was clear that Lee was the uncommitted partner and Jenna was the committed counterpart.

### Genogram

Lee was an only child from an upper-class family. His father was a high-level corporate executive as was his father before him. Lee claimed that he was not spoiled as a child, but his parents could easily afford to give him whatever he needed. The family belonged to an exclusive country club that his parents seemed to love and a vacation home in another country that had been passed down through the generations. Lee called his childhood "great." He said his younger sister felt the same way.

Lee excelled in both golf, tennis, and squash – which was important to his parents – and he had lots of friends in high school. He also had a "sweet girlfriend" from a fine family that his parents approved of. Lee followed high school by taking his father's advice and attending and graduating from the same expensive, private college his father went to. When I asked Lee about this, he said that he always knew he would go into a profession that focused on making money. And because his father was so successful, he trusted his dad to choose the right college for him, even if it was his father's alma mater. "If it was good enough for him, it was good enough for me," Lee said. Lee's sister also went to an exclusive college and married a wealthy man.

Lee had great admiration for his parents. He saw them as smart and attractive. He admitted that he enjoyed the privileged lifestyle he was raised in and wished to replicate it. Lee already belonged to his father's exclusive golf club and was close to buying his own vacation home. He said that he could easily ask his parents for the money, but he wanted to do this on his own. As mentioned, Lee made it a point to tell me that his parents did not think Jenna was good enough for him and warned him not to marry her.

Lee called his father a nice, fun-loving man, who worshipped his wife. Lee also saw him as a great guy to have a beer with if the conversation was simple and positive. Apparently, his father did not like to talk about negative things. If something emotionally difficult came up, Lee said that his father would leave it to his wife to manage. Lee said that it was hard to tell how his father really felt about something or if he was going along with his wife out of loyalty or fear of consequences. He said his guess was that his parents shared the same values.

Lee's mother was the "star" of the family. Lee laughed when he said that he admired his father for even getting her to marry him. She was from a wealthy family and very accomplished in her own right. She completed both an undergraduate and a graduate degree in economics with honors from an Ivy League university, where she excelled on the golf team. She also belonged to the most popular sorority at college and was, then and now, considered a socialite. Lee looked up to her, and although he said that he felt loved, he did not like disappointing her. He said that his father seemed easier to please.

Jenna grew up in a close-knit but poor Italian family. Her father died when she was nine years old of a sudden heart attack, and she and her two younger sisters lived with their mother up until she married Lee. Jenna was not parentified, however. She reported that her mother was a "strong, independent woman" who found a way to support the family.

Jenna looked up to her mother. She saw her as easy to talk to but quick to get anxious. She said that her mother needed to be in control, and given the loss of her husband and her difficult financial situation, she also felt sorry for her. She did not date much after her husband died, and according to Jenna, she became "more serious." Jenna also described her mother as very accepting of Lee and his family even though she felt inferior to them at times.

Jenna had two long-term relationships in high school. She told me that she was "a one-man woman." She added that these early relationships were typical of her age but that both boys broke up with her for what she called vague reasons. She repeated the same dynamic in college with the exception that one of her two boyfriends cheated on her. Jenna seemed a bit confused about the breakups. She hypothesized that she may have come off as desperately wanting a relationship.

Jenna attended a state college, did extremely well, and starred in softball. She received her master's degree in human relations from the same college but only worked for a short period of time before she met Lee. From that point forward, Lee and Jenna were a couple. Jenna said Lee was generous and fun but always maintained an uncomfortable distance. She said that on some long weekends, rather than visit her, he preferred to stay with his college buddies. She also said her old boyfriends seemed more interested in sex than Lee did but attributed it to Lee's extensive social life and love of sports.

Neither Lee nor Jenna was abused. Jenna's family had no history of addictions, and although Lee's parents liked to drink, this was mostly reserved for social settings. He said that he would see his parents "a little tipsy," especially at some country club gatherings, but nothing unmanageable. There were no paraphilias or fetishes reported, and both partners denied any affairs. Lee was not on medication, but Jenna took a low-dose antidepressant. She claimed that she was worried about her relationship and sensed Lee pulling further and further away.

### Assessment Summary

Lee was in conflict about his commitment to Jenna. He usually followed his parents' recommendations, but this time he failed to and married a woman they disapproved of. Lee liked Jenna and found her supportive but, in retrospect, admitted that his parents were right in that she was not his or his family's type. "She doesn't even dress the part," he said. Lee said that he initially did not intend to stay with Jenna in the long term. But as the years passed, he found it more difficult to leave her. He said he felt obligated and could not bear hurting her even though his increasingly distant, short-tempered behavior and regular criticisms of her were doing just that. He put her down in cruel ways at every turn. He, at times, played the sadist to her masochist.

Lee was never very attracted to Jenna, and although he thought she was a great person, he said that his type was a woman like his mother and sister – socialites who spent their days playing tennis and golf and engaging with other wealthy people at their country club. Because of Lee's lack of commitment, the couple had little to no passion, sex, and intimacy in their marriage.

Lee could not decide whether to stay and suffer with Jenna or to hurt her by ending their relationship. I found this conflict with commitment consistent with Lee's upbringing. Lee was planning to have a short-lived relationship or fling with Jenna and to eventually follow his parents' path. He rarely disagreed with them or challenged them, especially that of his mother's. But because he was a rule follower and a pleaser of women, he also had difficulty ending a marriage even if sanctioned to do so by his parents.

Jenna had a history of men who abandoned her, beginning with her beloved father. In high school and college, she would reveal her desperate need to form a long-term relationship only to scare many of her suitors off. I believe that she was also unconsciously replicating her fear of picking a dedicated man for fear he, too, might disappear. Jenna's conflict with commitment manifested in her history of choosing men who did not want the same commitment as she did. In a paradoxical way, she was demonstrating her own problem with commitment that was related to her fear of being without a man and being with one whom she could possibly lose. By choosing men with commitment issues, she would never be able to get control over her own conflict with commitment.

### Clinical Recommendations

Each partner must recognize and take responsibility for conflict a with commitment. Lee needed to acknowledge his difficulty differentiating from his parents. Specifically, he needed to better understand his powerful mother's influence and whether he wanted to end his relationship with Jenna because he is unhappy with her or because she does not meet his mother's standards. Only after he makes this decision can he decide whether he wants to fully commit to Jenna or not.

Jenna needs to recognize how her father's death left her with a void that she has been trying to fill but at the same time is afraid to do so, for fear of more potential loss. If she cannot take a risk, she will end up choosing men who are equally ambivalent about committing to her and her relationships will lack durability. This insight should help her to decide what to do with Lee and, at the very least, help her cope with any potential abandonment.

### Assessing Krish and Devi (See Figure 5.4)

Krish was a 24-year-old engineer who also held a master's degree in engineering management. Devi was a 23-year-old computer programmer.

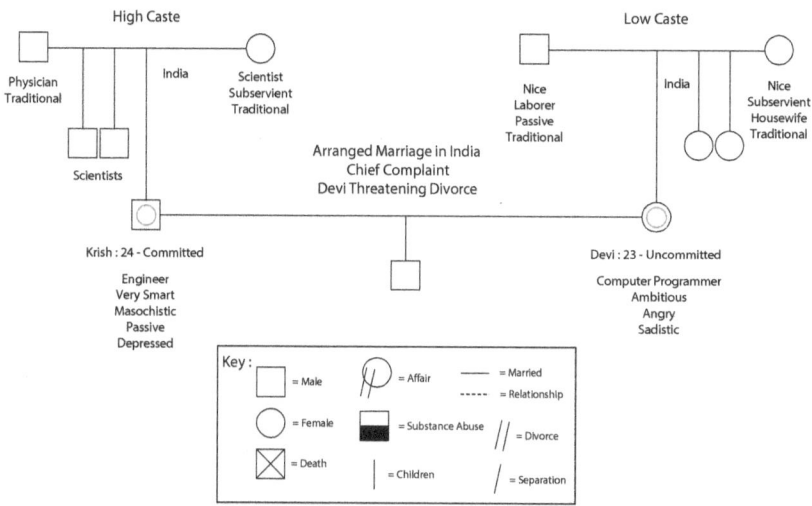

*Figure 5.4* Krish and Devi.

The couple were married in India, which both sets of parents arranged. Krish was from a higher caste than Devi, whose parents were very excited that their daughter was improving her station in life. The couple moved to the United States for Krish to attend graduate school at a prestigious university. Krish always finished at the top of his class and was thought to have great potential. The couple had been married for four years and had one young son.

### Initial Contact

Krish called to set up an appointment for him and Devi. He sounded anxious. He said that Devi is very angry and disappointed with him because he has not lived up to his potential. Apparently, she found him lazy. Devi was also tired of living in a small apartment, which is all the couple could afford. Unless Krish found a way to get promoted or to make more money, she said that she would probably leave him. Krish took his wife's threat seriously. He said that she has already stopped having sex with him and that she constantly ridicules almost every decision he makes.

### First Session

Krish was right; Devi was very angry with him. She claimed that he is a low achiever and that compared with his two older brothers and father, he was a "loser." Devi said that their marriage was arranged in India, and she agreed to it out of pressure from her parents and the community. But once the couple came to the United States, she felt free to express how she was feeling.

Devi was not only mad at Krish but all those involved in selecting the pair. This would include both sets of parents and their community in India. When she wasn't yelling at Krish, she was ignoring him. Although Devi had her doubts about the union, she thought that because Krish came from a higher caste and more successful family, he would catch up to others and surpass them.

Krish was a shy, quiet man raised in India. As mentioned, he came to the United States for a graduate degree, which he did obtain. He agreed that he was not earning as much as some of his colleagues but resented that Devi made it sound as if he was useless. He said that he saw no reason to overwork oneself just for money when they have enough to exist on. This kind of talk would enrage Devi, who wanted more out of life.

Krish said he was in love with Devi and found her physically attractive. He added that he was very hurt that she would not have sex with him and hoped that she could learn to respect him. He also said that he would be embarrassed if she left him.

I got the impression that Krish was under enormous pressure and that he might project onto the treatment process. Devi did seem to have a foot out the door, and I was not sure how much time Krish and the therapy had to make an impact. It was evident that Krish played the role of the committed and Devi played the role of the uncommitted.

### Genogram

Krish was the youngest of three brothers. Of all of them, he was deemed to be the smartest and carried the greatest chance of success. Krish was stellar in school. He attended a prestigious college for engineering in India followed by a graduate school in an Ivy League college in the Unites States. But Krish claimed that his father put an enormous amount of pressure on him to succeed and, in the process, made him a "nervous wreck." At one point, Krish thought he was having a breakdown, but he rallied.

Krish was also from a high-caste family. His father was a physician, and his mother was a scientist as were his two older brothers. Although Krish's father did have a good reason to bank on Krish – his test scores were usually near perfect – Krish decided that he wanted to live a stress-free life and took a job at a small engineering firm that paid little. Krish's entire family was disappointed with him, especially Devi.

Krish was taking medication for depression and anxiety when he first reported for treatment; Devi saw this as a weakness. It seemed as if Krish was a stress avoider and did what he could to take the easy way out. He knew that Devi was from a lower caste system, and he admitted that he thought because of this she should not put pressure on him.

Although Krish was very smart, especially with numbers, he was not very social and was bullied in elementary and high school in India. He claimed that he had suffered from low self-esteem as long as he could remember. He said that his brothers respected his brilliance but not his social capabilities and saw him as a "nerd."

Devi came from a lower caste, the oldest of three sisters. She described her parents as very nice, humble people who were both laborers in India. She said that she loved her parents but that they annoyed and frustrated her because they considered their low status in Indian society their fate. Devi said that if you are uneducated and poor in India, then you are subject to class discrimination.

Devi was the first on both sides of her extended family to go to college. She admitted that her goal was to achieve and to lift her status. She said that she thought Krish would help her to reach this goal; he was potentially a ticket to a better life. Devi claimed that she was by far the most attractive girl in her town in India, who could have gotten any man in her caste to marry her. But, because she wanted more from life, she chose to approve a marriage to Krish.

### Assessment Summary

Krish played the role of the committed, masochistic partner and Devi, the uncommitted sadistic partner. Krish defended what his wife called his laziness with the excuse that they did not need the money that badly and he preferred not to overwork. In essence, Krish was criticizing Devi's ambitiousness and alluding to it as neurotic. Devi was enraged with Krish. She distanced and stopped all sex, and there was no affection, passion, or intimacy in the relationship. Devi said she would leave the marriage unless Krish changed. Although Krish was annoyed by Devi, he did not want to lose her. While he was concerned about how a divorce would be perceived by his parents and community, Devi was not. She was mad at all who arranged the marriage, even herself.

Devi was in conflict about her commitment to Krish. She saw him as an avenue to the upper class and wanted to give Krish time to change. But she also did not think he was willing or capable of this change. Krish was tired of Devi and her demanding behavior. He saw her as bullying and materialistic. He described her as needlessly sadistic at times, even humiliating him in public. He did not think Devi ever loved him. But he was very attracted to her and did not think he could do any better. He also wanted to honor the arranged marriage and said he would feel embarrassed if Devi left him. Krish had low self-esteem and could not let go of Devi, but he nevertheless did not want to sacrifice his values for her. This was a good example of a transactional marriage.

*Clinical Recommendations*

Devi sanctioned the marriage arrangement to Krish only because she wanted a better life. She was not in love with or attracted to Krish physically. In fact, she found him boring and lazy. If Devi truly wanted to move up in class, she would then need to decide whether living in a loveless marriage was worth it. If not, she might need to end the relationship rather than stay and torture her husband. If Krish wanted Devi bad enough, he needed to decide whether he should show a little more ambition or let her go. Neither partner will get all that they want from each other, but if they can compromise, they may be able to stay together. How loving the relationship would be would depend on whether the two can accept new terms of the union.

### Assessing Thomas and Janie (See Figure 5.5)

Janie and Thomas were in their middle 30s and had three young children. Janie was a certified public accountant for a small firm and Thomas was a kindergarten teacher. The couple had been married for 12 years.

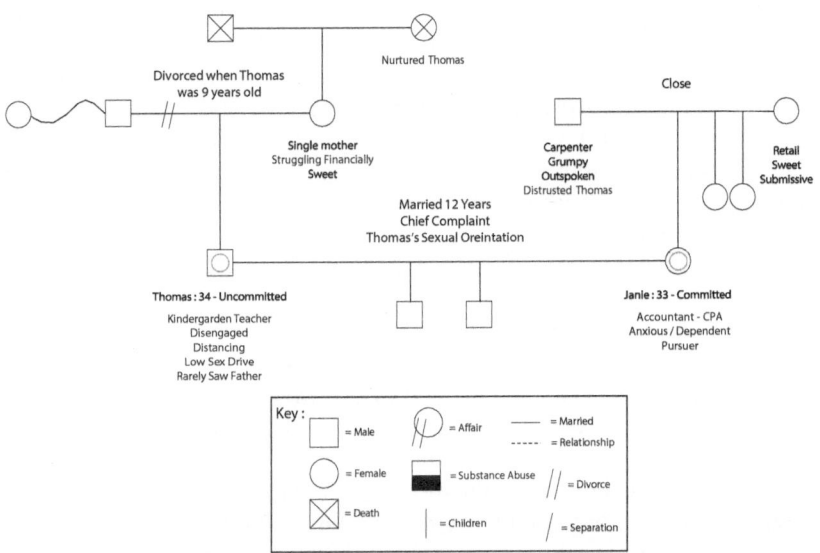

*Figure 5.5* Thomas and Janie.

### Initial Contact

Janie made the call for couples therapy. She said that Thomas was willing to go with her but was "scared to death." She claimed that he was a sweet man and a great father to their three children, but he was a conflict avoider. She also said he was shy and quiet. Janie said it was her idea to seek treatment because their once great sex life had dwindled and that although she is still very much in love with and attracted to Thomas, he no longer seems interested in her. She said she was hurt and confused. She hoped that Thomas could figure some things out in treatment.

### First Session

Thomas presented as a shy person. He looked extremely anxious and even seemed to stutter when answering some of my questions. Janie, on the contrary, was an energetic, vivacious personality. She found it easy to laugh and was as kind and gentle as Thomas. Both partners were careful not to criticize each other and held hands during the session.

When I asked why the couple sought treatment, Janie reiterated what she told me in our first contact. She felt Thomas slipping away from her and was not sure what was going on. She did not suspect him of an affair but there once great sex life had disappeared. She added that when she attempted to discuss the situation with Thomas, he seemed as confused about his behavior as she was. Janie said that although she was hurt, she felt sorry for Thomas. Other than that, she said that Thomas still treated her and the children as good as ever.

Thomas did seem confused. He claimed that his desire for Janie "just disappeared," although he did not find Janie any less physically attractive. He said that he loved his wife and felt she was a great companion. Apparently, Thomas did consult a urologist and was cleared of any organic issues. The physician found his testosterone to be normal and recommended couples/sex therapy. Thomas procrastinated in seeking treatment and so Janie took over and made the appointment. I suspected that Thomas was withholding something, but rather than press him, I proceeded to take a history.

### Genogram

Janie was the oldest of three sisters. She was a college graduate and worked long hours. Because her family was very close, she had built-in childcare. Janie claimed that her father was a master carpenter and her mother worked part-time in retail for a clothing store. She described her mother as sweet and supportive but subservient to her husband. Janie portrayed her father as a nice man but "a little rough around the edges." She said that she loved him, and they had always been close, but he was more conservative than she would have liked. She added that her father was upset when she broke up with a long-term boyfriend to date Thomas. He thought that there was something wrong with Thomas, but he did not know what. Janie said this annoyed her, but the best way to handle her father was to ignore him. Janie did not have a history of sexual problems, experienced orgasm, and said that Thomas was the best lover she ever had. She called him a giving, gentle lover who was always in touch with her needs.

Thomas was an only child. His parents divorced when he was nine years old, and he lived with his mother and maternal grandmother. He rarely saw his father after the divorce as his father moved several states away and took up residence with another woman whom Thomas knew very little about.

Thomas described his mother as a nice woman who was too busy struggling to make ends meet financially to pay much attention to him. He said that he got most of his nurturing from his grandmother, but she could not relate to him given her age. Although Thomas was not happy about his childhood, he said that he did not blame his mother. He said that he felt sorry for her and that he did his best to help her. He did not like or respect his father. He said he felt abandoned by him.

Thomas was not athletic in high school but studied hard and received good grades. He said the last thing his mother needed was for him to cause her more trouble. He went to community college and then transferred to a small state school and received his bachelor's degree in education. This is where he met Janie. The two have been together ever since.

Thomas had only one girlfriend before Janie. He claimed that she, like Janie, was very nice and fun-loving and that the only reason they broke up was because she chose to go to a college several states away. Thomas said that he understood why his girlfriend left but did feel abandoned by her. He said he probably would have married her if she had stayed.

Thomas claimed that he had no sexual problems with his ex-girlfriend. He was attracted to her and enjoyed having sex with her. The only other woman he had slept with was Janie. Thomas claimed that the main reason for his lack of partners over the years was his shyness. But Thomas did reveal something that Janie knew about – that he had slept with a few men before he met Janie. He said this was a pleasant experience but that he preferred to be straight. Oddly, Janie had little reaction to this, and when asked about it, she said that was all in the past and that "Thomas was probably just experimenting."

Neither partner had experienced any sexual abuse in their childhoods, and neither had any family members with substance abuse problems. Thomas had recently been prescribed medication for anxiety, and Janie suffered from stomach problems and chronic headaches, which she attributed to her job. Neither could pinpoint anything else they were upset about other than the presenting problem. Thomas did say that he hated making Janie feel bad, but he could not help it and at times felt as if he should just leave for the good of both.

### Assessment Summary

Janie was playing the role of the committed, anxious/dependent partner, and Thomas was playing the role of the uncommitted, distancing partner. He distanced from Janie, and he seemed distracted. Janie was still very attracted to Thomas and wanted desperately to help him any way she could. She does not want to give up on her marriage and prove her father correct about Thomas. She chose Thomas in part because she was trying to find a man who was different than her father – a kinder, gentler man. She chose a man whom she could talk to and who was very giving sexually. But Janie unconsciously chose a man who had experience in the gay world and might be considering a return to it.

Thomas loved Jamie and the life they had together. He has always wanted to be a tough guy, but he needed to decide his sexual orientation. He too did not want to prove Jamie's father right, but he could no longer stay in the relationship. His commitment problem was beginning to show serious symptoms via his emotional and sexual distancing. He was no longer the intimate partner Jamie claimed to crave.

### Clinical Recommendations

If Thomas was gay, Jamie needed to accept his true self and move on regardless of what her father thought. She needed to realize that she could find a caring, gentle straight man to meet her needs and to form a durable committed relationship with. Thomas needed to own his true self, whatever that was, rather than try to be someone he was not. To do so he might have to confront his homophobia so that he could truly commit to an appropriate partner and to form a stable and durable relationship.

## References

Abrams, J. A., Maxwell, M. L., & Belgrave, F. Z. (2018). Circumstances beyond their control: Black women's perceptions of black manhood. *Sex Roles, 79,* 151–162. https://doi.org/10.1007/s11199-017-0870–8

Aman, J., Abbas, J., Lela, U., & Shi, G. (2021). Religious factors promote marital commitment among married couples: Does religiosity help people amid religious affiliation, daily spirituals, and private the COVID-19 crisis? *Frontiers in Psychology, 12,* 1–19, https://doi.org/10.3389/fpsyg.2021.657400

American Psychological Association (2021). Worsening mental health crisis pressures psychology workforce: 2021 COVID-19 Practitioner Survey. https://www.apa.org/pubs/reports/practitioner/covid-19-2021

Applebury, G. (2020). What is reciprocity in romantic relationships? *Love to Know*. https://www.lovetoknow.com/life/relationships/what-is-reciprocity-romantic-relationship

Balderrama-Durbin, C. M., Fisette, K. L., & Synder, D. K. (2016). Best practices in assessment for couple therapy. In K. T. Sullivan & E. Lawrence (Eds.), *The Oxford handbook of relationship science and couple interventions* (pp. 131–147). Oxford University Press.

Barkley, S., & Tartakovsky, M. (2023). What to do if your partner doesn't want to attend marriage counseling. *PsychCentral*. https://psychcentral.com/relationships/what-to-do-when-your-partner-doesnt-want-to-attend-couples-counseling

Ben-Zeév, A. (2019). Friendship and romantic love. *Psychology Today*. https://www.psychologytoday.com/intl/blog/in-the-name-love/201908/friendship-and-romantic-love

Bergman, A. (2024). Gambling addiction statistics & facts 2024. *QuitGamble.com*. https://quitgamble.com/gambling-addiction-statistics-and-facts/

Berman, E. (1982). The individual interview as a treatment technique in conjoint therapy. *American Journal of Family Therapy, 10*, 27–37. https://doi.org/10.1080/01921.188268250434

Betchen, S. (2010). *Magnetic partners: Discover how the hidden conflict that once attracted to each other is now driving you apart*. Free Press.

Betchen, S. (2013, July). The slippery slope of open marriage. *Psychology Today*. https://www.psychologytoday.com/us/blog/magnetic-partners/201307/the-slippery-slope-open-marriage

Betchen, S. (2020, October). The importance of shared interests in relationships. *Psychology Today*. https://www.psychologytoday.com/us/blog/magnetic-partners/202010/the-importance-shared-interests-in-relationships

Betchen, S. (2022). *Couples in conflict: Clinical techniques for navigating sexual relationship control struggles*. Routledge.

Betchen, S. (2024). *Unmet expectations in couple and sex therapy: Helping couples negotiate realistic relationships*. Routledge.

Betchen, S., & Davidson, H. (2018). *Master conflict therapy: A new model for practicing couples and sex therapy*. Routledge.

Blum, A. (2024). Gay men in open relationships: What works? *Gay Therapy Center*. https://www.thegaytherapycenter.com/gay-men-in-open-relationships-what-works/

Booth, J. (2024). Dating statistics and facts 2024. *Forbes Health*. https://www.forbes.com/health/dating/dating-statistics/

Bowen, M. (1978). *Family therapy in clinical practice*. Aronson.

Braun-Harvey, D., & Vigorito, M. A. (2015). *Treating out of control sexual behavior: Rethinking sex addiction*. Springer.

Briggs-Gowan, M. J., Greene, C., Ford, J., Clark, R., McCarthy, K. J., & Carter, A. S. (2019). Adverse impact of multiple separations or loss of primary caregivers on young children. *European Journal of Psychotraumatology, 10*, 1–14. https://doi.org/10.1080/20008198.2019.1646965

Brogaard, B. (2015). 10 signs that your lover is commitment phobic. *Psychology Today*. https://www.psychologytoday.com/intl/blog/the-mysteries-of-love/201503/10-signs-that-your-lover-is-commitment-phobic

Call, V. R., & Heaton, T. B. (1997). Religious influence on marital stability. *Journal of the Scientific Study of Religion, 36*, 382–392. https://doi.org/10.2307/1387856

Collins, T. (2023). Why an addict can't love you: The battle between addiction and affection. *Faith Recovery Center.* https://www.faithrecoverybh.com/blog/why-an-addict-cant-love-you-the-battle-between-addiction-and-affection

Collisson, B. (2022). Interfaith relationships are becoming common: Do they work? *Psychology Today.* https://www.psychologytoday.com/us/blog/dating-toxic-or-tender/202210/interfaith-relationships-are-becoming-common-do-they-work

Dailey, R. M., Pfiester, A., Jin, B., Beck, G., & Clark, G. (2009). On-again/off-again dating relationships: How are they different from other dating relationships? *Personal Relationships, 16*, 23–47. https://doi.org/10.1111/j.1475-6811.2009.01208.x

DeMaria, R., Weeks, G., & Twist, M. (2017). *Focused genograms: Intergenerational assessment of individuals, couple, and families* (2nd ed.). Routledge.

Doherty, W. J. (2002). How therapists harm marriages and what we can do about it. *Journal of Couple & Relationship Therapy, 1*, 1–17. https://doi.org/10.1300/J398v01n02_01

Doherty, W. J., Harris, S. M., Hall, E. L., & Hubbard, A. K. (2021). How long do people wait before seeking couples therapy: A research note. *Journal of Marital and Family Therapy, 47*, 882–890. https://doi.org/10.1111/jmft.12479.

Francis-Tan, A., & Mialon, H. M. (2015). "A diamond is forever" and other fairy tales: The relationship between wedding expenses and marriage duration. *Economic Inquiry, 53*, 1919–1930. https://doi.org/10.1111/ecin.12206

Gambescia, N., Weeks, G., & Hertlein, K. (2021). The sexual genogram in assessment. In K. Hertlein, G. Weeks, & N. Gambescia (Eds.), *A clinician's guide to systemic sex therapy* (3rd ed.). Routledge.

Gaspard, T. (2024). Timing is everything when it comes to marriage counseling. *The Gottman Institute.* https://www.gottman.com/blog/timing-is-everything-when-it-comes-to-marriage-counseling/

Gillette, H. (2022). The four stages of the cycle of abuse: From tension to calm and back. *PsychCentral.* https://psychcentral.com/health/cycle-of-abuse#stages-of-the-cycle-of-abuse

George, M. B. (2024). What does trust and commitment look like in a relationship. *The Gottman Institute.* https://www.gottman.com/blog/what-does-trust-and-commitment-look-like-in-a-relationship/

Gleeson, B. (2022, November). Does society have a sex addiction problem? *The Mayo Clinic Health System.* https://www.mayoclinichealthsystem.org/hometown-health/speaking-of-health/does-society-have-a-sex-addiction-problem

Gottman, J., & Gottman, J. (2024). Enhanced Gottman relationship checkup. *The Questionnaire.* https://www.checkup.gottman.com

Gunther, R. (2011). Promise keepers – The committed partners who stay faithful to each other. *Psychology Today.* https://www.psychologytoday.com/us/blog/rediscovering-love/201112/promise-keepers-the-committed-partners-who-stay-faithful-each-other

Gupta, S., Tarantino, M., & Sanner, C. (2023). A scoping review of research on polyamory and consensual nonmonogamy: Implications for a more inclusive family science. *Journal of Family Theory & Review*, 1–40. https://doi.org/10.1111/jftr.12546

Hakkim, S., Yasir Arafat, S. M., Mahmud, I., Sathian, B., Sivasubramanian, M., & Kabir, R. (2022). Pornography – Is it good for sexual health? A systemic review. *Journal of Psychosexual Health, 4*, 111–122. https://doi.org/10.1177/26318318221088949

Heitler, S. (2022). Can relationships improve when just one partner gets help? *Psychology Today*. https://www.psychologytoday.com/us/blog/resolution-not-conflict/202210/can-relationships-improve-when-just-one-partner-gets-help

Hendrick, S. S., Dicke, A., & Hendrick, C. (1998). The Relationship Assessment Scale. *Journal of Social and Personal Relationships, 15*, 137–152. https://doi.org/10.1177/0265407598151009

Herrero, J., Torres, A., & Rodriguez-Diaz, F. J. (2018). Child abuse, risk in male patient selection, and intimate partner violence victimization of women of the European union. *Prevention Science, 19*, 1102–1112. https://doi.org/10.1007/s11121-018-0911-8

Herzberg, B. (2023). 5 Reasons why a partner might refuse couples therapy. *Psychology Today*. https://www.psychologytoday.com/us/blog/the-psychology-of-relationships-and-emotional-intelligence/202310/5-reasons-why-your-partner

Horowitz, J., Graf, N., & Livingston, G. (2019). Marriage and cohabitation in the U.S. *Pew Research Center*. https://www.pewresearch.org/social-trends/2019/11/06/marriage-and-cohabitation-in-the-u-s/

Jacobsen, J. (2023). 22 signs you are dating a commitment phobe. *Marriage.com*. https://www.marriage.com/advice/relationship/dating-a-commitment-phobe/

Joyner, K., Manning, W., & Prince, B. (2019). The qualities of seme-sex and different-sex Couples. *Journal of Marriage and Family, 81*, 487–505. https://doi.org/10.1111/jomf.12535.

Kanngiesser, P., Serko, D., & Woike, J. K. (2023). Promises on the go: A field study on keeping one's word. *Frontiers in Psychology, 14*, 1–7. https://doi.org/10.3389/fpsy.2023.1097239

Kelberga, A., & Martinsone, B. (2021). Differences in motivation to engage in sexual activity between people in monogamous and non-monogamous committed relationships. *Frontiers in Psychology, 12*. https://doi.org/10.3389/fpsyg.2021.753460

Khalifian, C. E., Barry, R. A. (2020). Expanding intimacy theory: Vulnerable disclosures and partner responding. *Journal of Social and Personal Relationships, 37*, 58–76. https://doi.org/10.1177/0265407519853047

Kogan, S., Yu, T., & Brown, L. G. (2016). Romantic relationship commitment behavior among emerging adult African American men. *Journal of Marriage and Family, 78*, 996–1012. https://doi.org/10.1111/jomf.12293

Kohut, T., Balzarini, R. N., Rogge, R. D., Shaw, A. M., McNulty, J. K., Russell, V. M., Fisher, W. A., & Campbell, L. (2021). But what's your partner up to? Associations between relationship quality and pornography use depend on contextual patterns of use within the couple. *Journal of Social and Personal Relationships, 35*, 655–676. https://doi.org/10.3389/fpsyg.2021.661347

Leone, C. (2023). Individual sessions as part of couples therapy? How concepts from self psychology can help us decide. *Psychoanalysis, Self and Context, 18*, 218–233. https://doi.org/10.1080/24720038.2023.2184821

Levine, E. C., Herbenick, D., Martinez, O., Fu, T. C., & Dodge, B. (2018). Nonconsensual nonmonogamy, and monogamy among U. S. adults: Findings from the 2012 National Survey of Sexual Health and Behavior. Archives of Sexual Behavior, 47, 1439–1450. https://doi.org/10.1007/s10508-018-1178-7.

Mandriota, M. (2021). Here is how to identify your attachment style. PsychCentral. https://psychcentral.com/health/4-attachment-styles-in-relationships

Marie, S. (2021). What to do if your partner won't consider couples therapy. Healthline. https://www.healthline.com/health/relationships/partner-wont-consider-couples-therapy

Martin, S. (2018). Why do we repeat the same dysfunctional relationship patterns over and over? PsychCentral. https://psychcentral.com/blog/imperfect/2018/07/why-do-we-repeat-the-same-dysfunctional-relationship-patterns

McHale, S. M., Updegraff, K. A., & Whiteman, S. D. (2012). Sibling relationships and influences in childhood and adolescence. Journal of Marriage and Family, 74, 913–930. https://doi.org/10.1111/j.1741-3737.2012.01011.x

Mernitz, S. E. (2018). A cohort comparison of trends in first cohabitation duration in the United States. Demographic Research, 38, 2071–2086. https://doi.org/10.4054/DemRes.2018.38.66

Moors, A. C., Gesselman, A. N., & Garcia, J. R. (2021). Five misconceptions about consensually nonmonogamous relationships. Current Directions in Psychological Science, 32, 355–361. https://doi.org/10.1177/09637214231166853

Morin, A. (2024). How parents fighting could affect a child's mental health. Verywellfamily. https://www.verywellfamily.com/how-parents-fighting-affects-children-s-mental-health-4158375

Negash, S., & Morgan, M. (2016). A family affair: Examining the impact of parental infidelity on children using a structural family therapy framework. Contemporary Family Therapy, 38. 1–13, https://doi.org/10.1007/s1059-015-9364-4

Office for National Statistics (2017). People who were abused as children are more likely to be abused as an adult. Data and Analysis for Census 2021. https://www.ons.gov.uk/peoplepopulationandcommunity/crimeandjustice/articles/peoplewhowereabusedaschildrenaremorelikelytobeabusedasanadult/2017-09-27

Pew Research Center (2015). America's changing religious landscape. https://www.pewresearch.org/religion/2015/05/12/americas-changing-religious-landscape/

Rhoades, G. K., Stanley, S. M., Markman, H., & Ragan, E. P. (2012). Parents' marital status, conflict, and role modeling: Links with adult romantic relationship quality. Journal of Divorce & Remarriage, 53, 348–367. https://doi.org/10.1080%2F10502556.2012.675838

Ritchie, L. L., Knopp, K., & Rhoades, G. K. (2019). Assessment in couple and family therapy. In J. Lebow, A. L. Chambers, & D. C. Breulin (Eds.), Encyclopedia in couples and family therapy (pp. 144–148). Springer.

Rodman, S. (2018). Commitment issues: 11 signs & how to deal with them. https://www.talkspace.com/blog/commitment-issues-reasons/

Rosenfeld, M. J., Thomas, R. J., & Hausen, S. (2019). Disintermediating your friends: How online dating in the United States displaces other ways of meeting. Proceedings of the National Academy of Sciences (PNAS), 116, 17753–17758. https://doi.org/10.1073/pnas.1908630116

Rostosky, S. S., Riggle, E. D. B., Dudley, M. G., & Wright, M. L. C. (2006). Commitment in same-sex relationships: A qualitative analysis of couples' conversions. *Journal of Homosexuality, 51*, 199–222. https://doi.org/10.1300/j082v51n03_10

Schechinger, H. A., Sakuluk, J. K., & Moors, A. C. (2018). Harmful and helpful therapy practices with consensually non-monogamous clients: Toward an inclusive framework. *Journal of Consulting and Clinical Psychology, 86*, 879–891. https://doi.org/10.1037/ccp0000349

Selterman, D., Garcia, J. R., & Tsapelas, I. (2019). Motivations of extradyadic infidelity Revisited. *Journal of Sex Research, 56*, 273–286. https://doi.org/10.1080/00224499.2017.1393494

Stanley, S. M., & Rhoades, G. K. (2023). What's the plan? Cohabitation, engagement, and divorce. Institute for Family Studies. https://ifstudies.org/ifs-admin/resources/reports/cohabitationreportapr2023-final.pdf

Stewart-Williams, S., Butler, C. A., & Thomas, A. G. (2017). Sexual history and present attractiveness: People want a mate with a bit of a past, but not too much. *Journal of Sex Research, 54*, 1097–1105. https://doi.org/10.1080/00224499.2016.1232690

Strauss-Cohen, I. (2023). 6 truths about people who go to therapy. *Psychology Today*. https://www.psychologytoday.com/ca/blog/your-emotional-meter/202307/the-truth-about-people-who-go-to-therapy

Sullivan, K. T. (2001). Understanding the relationship between religiosity and marriage: An investigation of the immediate and longitudinal effects of religiosity on newlywed couples. *Journal of Family Psychology. 15*, 610–626. https://doi.org/10.1037/0893-3200.15.4.610

Tahir, N. N. (2021). Understanding arranged marriage: An unbiased analysis of a traditional marital institution. *International Journal of Law, Policy and the Family, 35*, 1–20. https://doi.org/10.1093/lawfam/ebab005

U.S. Department of Health and Human Services (HHS) (2023). Substance abuse and mental health services administration (SAMHSA). Release 2022 National Survey on Drug Use and Health Data. https://www.samhsa.gov/newsroom/press-announcements/20231113/hhs-samhsa-release-2022-nsduh-data

Vennum, A., Lindstrom, R., Monk, J. K., & Adams, R. (2014). It's complicated: The continuity and correlates of cycling in cohabitating and marital relationships. *Journal of Social and Personal Relationships, 31*, 410–430. https://doi.org/10.1177/0265407513501987

Vogels, E. A. & McClain, C. (2023). Key findings about online dating in the U.S. Pew Research Center. https://www.pewresearch.org/short-reads/2023/02/02/key-findings-about-online-dating-in-the-u-s/

Weeks, G., & Fife, S. (2014). *Couples in treatment: Techniques and approaches for effective practice* (3rd ed.). Routledge.

Weiss, R. (2020). The consequences of compulsive porn use. *PsychCentral*. https://psychcentral.com/blog/sex/2020/07/the-consequences-of-compulsive-porn-use#1

Wheatley Institute (2021). Brigham Young University. National couples and pornography survey 2021. *National Couples and Pornography Survey 2021*. https://wheatley.byu.edu/national-couples-and-pornography-survey-2021

Wilcox, B., Dew, J., & Elhage, E. (2019). Institute for Family Studies. Cohabitation doesn't compare: Marriage, cohabitation, and relationship quality. *Institute for Family Studies*. https://ifstudies.org/blog/cohabitation-doesnt-compare-marriage-cohabitation-and-relationship-quality

Wiley, J., Wilkinson, I., & Young, L. (2005). [Database record]. APA PsycTests. https://doi.org/10.1037/t11931-000

Winston, S. (2018). When someone has one foot out the door. *Psychology Today*. https://www.psychologytoday.com/intl/blog/shift-happens/201809/when-someone-has-one-foot-out-the-door

Wolfinger, N. H. (2018). Does sexual history affect marital happiness? *Institute for Family Studies*. https://ifstudies.org/blog/does-sexual-history-affect-marital-happiness

World Population Review (2024). Arranged marriage countries 2024. https://worldpopulationreview.com/country-rankings/arranged-marriage-countries

# Clinical Treatment of Romantic Commitment

# Chapter 6

# Treating Couples with Commitment Conflicts

The assessment phase naturally flows into the formal treatment process. And by the time this transition occurs, the therapist should be able to identify the couple's interactional style, determine if the couple suffer from an unbalanced conflict with commitment, and reveal the origin of the conflict. Simply put, a solid clinical framework from which to begin the formal treatment process should be in place. The therapist should, however, remain open to new data no matter how much this new information contradicts the assessment and framework. While this model relies heavily on therapist insight and observation to assess a couple, the couple's feedback is considered vital (Reese et al., 2010). True assessment never ends until the couple terminates treatment.

The conflict approach, previously applied to control struggles and unmet expectations in couples (Betchen, 2022, 2024), is modified to treat romantic relationships with symptoms resulting from a conflict with commitment. The treatment process is a multi-layered approach that consists of the following seven clinical steps:

*Step 1. Determine the couple's interactional process or committed–uncommitted dynamic and how it enables the couple's symptoms in the context of attachment, love, intimacy, and passion.*
*Step 2. Expose the couple's internalized shared conflict with commitment and how each partner colludes in maintaining it.*
*Step 3. Demonstrate how mate choice is based on the couple's shared conflict.*
*Step 4. Broaden the couple's context beyond romantic commitment.*
*Step 5. Expose the origin of each partner's conflict.*
*Step 6. Help each partner to differentiate from their respective families of origin to balance the shared conflict and to gain more control over it.*
*Step 7. Alleviate commitment symptoms to develop a more durable relationship.*

DOI: 10.4324/9781003475743-9

While these steps may overlap during the treatment process, they do tend to build upon one another. Therefore, I recommend that the couples therapist move in sequence. In my teachings and supervision, trainees and supervisees are often so anxious to alleviate the couple's pain they act too quickly, failing to gather enough data on the couple. This may result in the therapist misunderstanding or misdiagnosing the couple.

## Clinical Case Examples

The following three cases are detailed accounts of how I utilize the seven-step treatment process with a variety of couples. Each case is a composite of two to three. Names, ages, and professions are changed to protect couple confidentiality. Brief vignettes are included. In this therapeutic process, the therapist weaves together the couple's symptom(s), interactional style, and their shared conflict with commitment. This process is necessary to balance the conflict and alleviate the couple's symptoms.

### Scott and Emma (See Figure 6.1)

Emma was a 42-year-old economics professor. Her live-in boyfriend, Scott, was a 44-year-old executive. The couple had no children together, but each

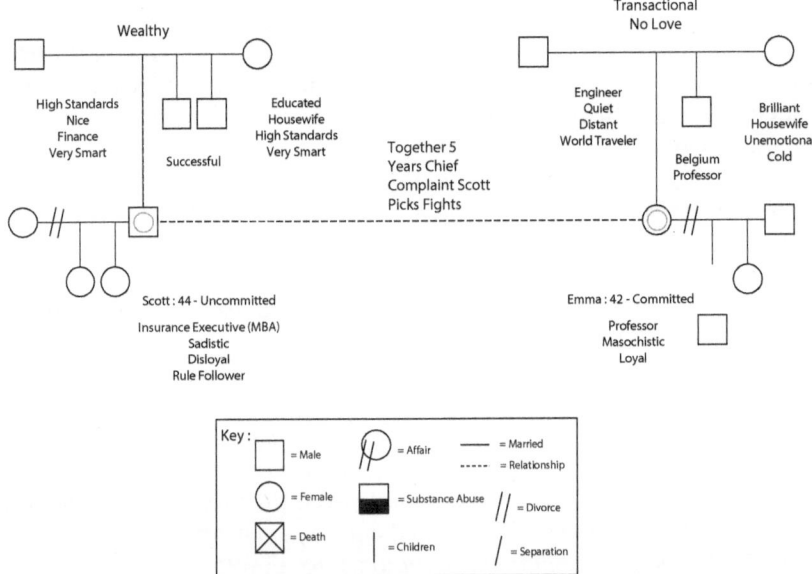

Figure 6.1 Scott and Emma.

had two from previous marriages. They had been living together for approximately five years at the time of treatment.

### Initial Contact

Emma made the initial call. She said that she and Scott were fighting and that he was often "mean" to her. She called him a "grump" who verbally attacks her every chance he gets. For example, Scott would criticize Emma's style of dress or rant at her about failing to keep the car's gas tank full.

Emma said that she is confused. She adores Scott and gives him all the sex and affection he wants. She said that she loves taking care of his needs, but that he always seems annoyed with her. "He makes me feel like I'm always in his way," she said. Emma does not know how to please Scott and she finds his behavior toward her depressing. According to Emma, Scott was resistant to couples therapy but acquiesced to quiet Emma.

### First Session

Scott was very angry with Emma, but he could not seem to identify what it was about her that made him so upset. He agreed that she was sexually open and willing to meet his needs, but still he was disgusted with her. Sometimes I would catch him almost sneering at her when she spoke. No doubt Scott was playing the role of the uncommitted partner and Emma agreed. "At times I feel as if he just wants to run away. I am worried that he is not 'all in,'" she said. I did not sense that Scott was cheating. Emma claimed that he was around all the time and that cheating was not her worry. But I did suspect that something deeper was afoot with Scott.

Emma presented just as she did in the initial contact – anxious. Although visibly upset with Scott's criticisms of her, she took them in and rarely went on the offensive. She believed that it would make him angrier and push him even further away. Emma struck me as somewhat needy and desperate to save her marriage. She still had high hopes of adopting a child with Scott. She clearly demonstrated a low self-worth and could not bring herself to entertain the thought of ending the relationship. Emma assumed the role of the committed partner in the relationship.

### Genogram

Emma was the oldest of two siblings – she had a younger brother. Emma's father was a quiet, distant man who traveled the world as a civil engineer. He had several patents and was described as brilliant. But he was rarely home and had little relationship with his children. Emma's brother sought his college education in France and settled in nearby Belgium. He was a professor of political science. Emma also studied overseas but came home to complete her graduate degrees and to start a career in academia.

Emma's mother was also described as brilliant. But she was both withholding and distant. According to Emma, her mother attended to her basic needs but was not one to show emotion. She saw little affection between her parents, and she felt as if her father could not wait to go away on business. Her mother rarely complained about this because Emma thought she too did not mind the distance. She was unclear as to whether her parents loved each other or were together out of habit and convenience.

Emma said that she did not date very much in high school or college, in part, because she was shy and lacked confidence. But she also preferred to put all her efforts into her education. She saw this as an avenue to impress her parents. But despite her academic achievements, Emma reported her parents offered no positive reinforcement. When she complained, her mother coldly responded, "You have your degrees, isn't that enough?" Emma claimed that the couple of boyfriends she had eventually cheated or broke up with her for someone else. She said her ex-husband did the same.

Emma reported no sexual difficulty and in fact claimed to enjoy sex even if she sometimes felt mistreated. She said that it made her feel good to please her boyfriends and she had hoped it would keep them around. Other than her parents' coldness, Emma reported no abuse. She took no medication, although she was considering something for her depression. There was no addictive behavior reported in Emma's family of origin.

Scott was the oldest of three brothers, all very successful. Scott got his master's in business administration (MBA) degree and worked his way up to the top of a large insurance company. He described his father as a nice man who made a fortune in the finance industry and held two Ivy League graduate degrees. He said that his mother also graduated from a prestigious school but settled for being a housewife.

Scott said that he was close to his parents, but they held high standards and had a lot of rules. He said that if you followed the rules, they were easy to get along with. If you rebelled, however, he said they would team up and "shun" you.

Scott was an admitted rule follower, and his parents made it known that they approved of Emma – they saw her as "their kind of person." That is, she was well educated and came from a good family. Scott said that they put pressure on him to continue to date her and warned him not to sabotage the relationship. They gave him the clear message that one needs to recognize a good thing and seize it rather than foolishly miss a great opportunity.

Scott believed that because his parents were so smart, they were rarely wrong. He claimed that every time he rebelled, he screwed up and would suffer the consequences. He also feared their shunning style of punishment. He said it made him feel like a "loser for embarrassing the family."

Scott dated frequently but was careful only to bring certain women home to meet his parents. The woman had to be smart, beautiful, ambitious, and from a cultured family. He claimed that there were many women whom he liked but was afraid to engage. He spoke of one woman he fell in love with but felt compelled to break up with her because he knew his parents would disapprove.

Shunning notwithstanding, Scott did not suffer any abuse growing up. He reported no history of sexual difficulty and no out-of-control sexual behavior. He performed well with Emma. Scott only took medication for his cholesterol. This was the couple's second stint in couples therapy. They said they learned some communication skills but, overall, Scott found it a waste of money. He stopped treatment despite a mild protest from Emma.

*Assessment Summary*

As mentioned, Scott played the role of the uncommitted, sadistic, disloyal partner and Emma played the role of the committed partner, masochistic, loyal partner. The symptoms of commitment were found to be in the areas of love and intimacy. Scott did not seem to love Emma, and he was certainly not in love with her. While the couple still had passionate sex, for Scott, this was purely a physical experience as Emma was a skilled lover.

Beyond sex, Scott and Emma were rarely intimate. When they did speak, Scott was usually critical of Emma and picked on her for everything, from the way she dressed to her decision-making ability. Emma admitted love for Scott even though she found him abusive at times. She said that although the way he treated her eroded some of her love for him, she still wanted to marry him. She wished she could be with him more.

Scott did not want to be with Emma. He was not in love with her and never was. But he was also a rule follower, and he almost always obliged his parents who saw Emma as a perfect match for him. If Scott followed his heart instead of his parents, he would have avoided most of the time spent with Emma and set her free to find someone who truly wanted her. Instead, he dated her for several years without having any desire to commit to her. And this low commitment was demonstrated on several levels given the couple's difficulties with love and intimacy – ingredients of a romantic commitment.

Scott witnessed his parents' transactional type of relationship and replicated it in real time. His parents were together primarily for class-related and financial reasons and not because they loved each other or liked to spend time together. They, too, were beholden to their own set of rules and values.

Scott was abusive and neglectful, but his behavior was not personal. Rather, it was a projection of the feelings he experienced as a trapped individual. Blaming his parents for his entrapment was far too dangerous, so he unconsciously chose to take his self-hatred and rage out on someone he perceived would tolerate it without leaving him. It was a sadistically brilliant maneuver because this way Scott could maintain distance from Emma and spare his parents simultaneously.

Emma was an intelligent woman, but she suffered from very low self-esteem and self-worth. Given her family of origin, it made sense that she would grow up with a longing to be loved and with feelings of unworthiness.

### Clinical Recommendations

Scott needed to admit to himself that he did not want to be with Emma. But to do so, he needed to differentiate enough from his parents and be true to his own needs. He also needed to recognize that he was striking out sadistically because he felt trapped. To achieve these objectives, Scott had to risk alienating his parents. As it stood, he was more committed to them than he was to Emma. This is Scott's conflict with commitment: He wanted to leave Emma but could not muster the strength and courage to do so. Instead, he remained trapped and tortured her. To balance this conflict with commitment and to establish a durable relationship, Scott needed to recognize that his parents were still in charge of his life.

Emma needed to realize that even though she wanted to save her relationship, she did not have the power to do so. Emma was desperate for love but conflicted about whether she deserved it. This fit with her experiences in her family of origin: cold, unloving parents enabled her to choose men who were equally cold to her and conflicted with commitment. It only looked as if Emma was more committed than Scott because she pursued him for commitment. Her conflict manifested in her ability to commit to a man who could not commit to her. Together the couple colluded in maintaining their unbalanced shared conflict and its resultant symptoms.

To balance her conflict with commitment and alleviate her symptoms, Emma needed to accept that her parents were neglectful and unloving and acknowledge how this affected her inability to be loved and committed to. She then needed to decide whether she wanted to allow others, like Scott, to treat her as her parents did or to allow herself to be loved and committed to.

### Treatment

**Step 1. Determine the couple's interactional process or committed–uncommitted dynamic and how it enables the couple's symptoms in the context of attachment, love, intimacy, and passion.**

Given the data collected from the initial contact, first session, and the genogram work, and through observation of the couple interaction, the therapist determined that Scott was playing the role of the uncommitted partner and Emma was playing the role of the committed partner. In the following vignette, the therapist made a connection between these roles and their symptoms with love and intimacy.

*Therapist:*  Scott, I can tell that you are not thrilled to be here.
*Scott:*  I think it's a waste of good money. I'm only doing this to shut Emma up.
*Therapist:*  So, you don't think that it can help your relationship?
*Scott:*  I don't know.
*Therapist:*  Do you want help with it?
*Scott:*  I'm not sure. I don't know if I want to stay in it.
*Therapist:*  You don't sound very committed.
*Scott:*  Yeah well…
*Therapist:*  Emma, how committed has Scott been acting?
*Emma:*  Like he's being held captive. And I do everything for him. I wash his clothes, cook his meals, and I give him all the sex he wants. In return I get yelled at and criticized. It's as if I can't do anything right. My friends see the way he treats me, and they think I should leave him.
*Therapist:*  You sound very unhappy. What keeps you from leaving?
*Emma:*  I love Scott. And I want to marry and start a family.
*Therapist:*  So, even though Scott doesn't share his life with you, you are committed enough to him to start a family?
*Emma:*  I'm all in, as they say.
*Therapist:*  How about you, Scott? Where are you at?
*Scott:*  I don't know. Emma is not a bad person, but I don't know where I am in this relationship.
*Therapist:*  Well, you haven't left either. What's holding you?
*Scott:*  I'm not sure. I know my parents would be upset if I left. They really like Emma. And it's not like Emma is a terrible person. She isn't. And sometimes I feel bad about the way I treat her. Other times I feel she deserves it.

### Step 2. Expose the couple's internalized shared conflict with commitment and how they collude in maintaining it.

*Therapist:*  I notice you both are unhappy with your current situation but see some value in maintaining it.
*Emma:*  Like I said, I love Scott and I want him to invest in our relationship.
*Therapist:*  But suppose he doesn't want to, or can't?
*Emma:*  Why wouldn't he?

*Therapist:*    I don't know. Why wouldn't you, Scott?

*Scott:*    I don't know.

*Therapist:*    But can you admit that you are not as invested in the relation-ship as Emma would like you to be?

*Scott:*    Yes. I admit that.

*Therapist:*    So, you are not fully committed to Emma, but do not want to do anything about it?

*Scott:*    I guess. I can't control my actions. Is that stupid?

*Therapist:*    Not really. But it does sound like you are conflicted about committing to her. And how about you Emma? You are un-happy but you won't leave. Your hope is that a man who is conflicted about committing to you will change. You sound like a gambling woman.

*Emma:*    I never saw myself that way.

*Therapist:*    Well, maybe you're conflicted about someone committing to you.

*Emma:*    I hope not. But I do have a history of dating men who are "play-ers" and do not seem interested in a long-term relationship.

### Step 3. Demonstrate how mate choice is based on this shared conflict.

*Therapist:*    Scott, it looks as if you are the trapped partner, but I suspect Emma is trapped as well.

*Emma:*    I don't feel trapped. I feel like I want to be here.

*Therapist:*    Do you know what I mean, Scott?

*Scott:*    Yes, I think so. Emma, how can you be happy with the way I treat you? Any sane person would have left by now. But you can't.

*Emma:*    I stay because I believe in love. I do want you to treat me bet-ter; that's why I'm here.

*Therapist:*    Emma, I do not doubt your love for Scott. But all the dedica-tion and commitment will not work with someone who cannot reciprocate. And Scott cannot seem to, nor does it look like he wants to. If it were not for you, would he be here right now? Would he have suggested getting help for this relationship? Would you have, Scott?

*Scott:*    (Looking downward) No.

*Therapist:*    What I am suggesting is that you both have the same conflict but that it manifests differently.

*Scott:*    My conflict shows in my mistreatment of Emma, and Emma puts up with it.

*Therapist:*    Right. Got it, Emma?

| Emma: | My friends and family put it differently. They think I'm pathetic for tolerating Scott. |
|---|---|
| Therapist: | Speaking in a nonsexual context, there does seem to be some sadomasochistic behavior involved. |

### Step 4. Broaden the couple's context beyond romantic commitment.

This step is not always needed for couples who accept that a shared conflict is operating and responsible for their relational symptoms. These couples are less defensive and thus easier to treat. But other couples hyper-focus on their specific symptoms in the context of their relationship only. And that is all they want to talk about. They may feel that the therapist is wasting their time or off-track if anything else is brought up. These couples contain their problems. This allows them to blame one another for their issues rather than accept the pervasiveness of their problem or that it may exist in other contexts as well. The following vignette will demonstrate this.

| Emma: | Scott is not just unhappy with me; he's generally miserable. He complains about the insurance industry all the time, and he hates the President of his company even though the guy promoted him. |
|---|---|
| Therapist: | What do you think about that Scott? |
| Scott: | I think I'm more miserable at home. |
| Therapist: | So, you think that Emma is the cause of all your misery? |
| Scott: | Maybe not Emma per se, but my feeling trapped might be. |
| Emma: | Did I just get a compliment? |
| Therapist: | So, you've never felt like this before, Scott? |
| Emma: | Scott feels trapped at work also. He's always complaining about the insurance industry and what he should have done differently with his life. |
| Scott: | Well, that's true. I am stuck there. |
| Emma: | I just thought of this, but he can't even let go of old friends who he can't stand. |
| Scott: | That's true. And you are mistreated at work. |
| Emma: | Yeah, I feel that way. I never made the connection. Maybe I have trouble taking care of and standing up for myself, with or without Scott. |

### Step 5. Expose the origin of each partner's conflict.

It is here that the couples therapist is met with the most resistance from the couple. Some partners are uncomfortable discussing their families of origin because it makes them feel as if they are blaming their parents for their relationship problems. These individuals would much rather blame one another than their parents. The following vignette will illustrate how the couples therapist can bypass some of these resistances.

*Therapist:*   We have been discussing your shared conflict with commitment but haven't addressed where it might come from.

*Scott:*   Do we need to know where it came from if we acknowledge its existence?

*Emma:*   I would like to know. I think your parents like to be in control, and you can't make up your own mind without their approval. And even when you don't take their advice, you are so tortured about disappointing them.

*Therapist:*   Scott, can you recall times that your parents disappointed you or made you angry?

*Scott:*   Does all that matter?

*Emma:*   He runs from a discussion like this. It looks like he's running again. He doesn't want to accept that his parents run his life. He can't acknowledge their manipulative ways. That's why we are here today.

*Therapist:*   Emma, are you suggesting that Scott's parents pushed him into this relationship and that he is in conflict about it?

*Emma:*   Something like that.

*Scott:*   (Sarcastic) Let's just blame our parents for everything that goes wrong with us. It's all their fault.

*Therapist:*   All I think Emma is trying to say is that part of you wants to please your parents and yet there might be another side that would rather make your own choices free of criticism. And, that this type of conflict can be responsible for your misery and your difficulty with commitment.

*Scott:*   I'll think about that one.

### Step 6. Help partners to differentiate from their respective families of origin to balance the shared conflict and to gain more control over it.

There is easily the most sophisticated part of the therapeutic process. It is the time when each partner must decide what to give up and what to keep. And not just on a physical level but on an emotional one as well. This is a time of confusion in part because whichever decision a partner makes, there will also be a loss associated with it.

*Therapist:*   Emma, you suggested that Scott is usually aligned with his parents.

*Emma:*   More like, "joined at the hip." Look, I'm not suggesting that all their decisions are bad, but we better be in line with them or else. But Scott will have to see this before he can do anything about it. He still doesn't get it.

Scott:        Suppose I don't want to do anything about it?

Therapist:    Well, I suspect you will stay stuck for the rest of your life.

Emma:        He's good at staying stuck.

Scott:        So, it's either me or them, right?

Therapist:    It's your call, Scott. If you do not think your parents continue to play a significant role in your conflict, you may not be able to negotiate a middle ground with your conflict.

Scott:        What does that have to do with my being stuck?

Therapist:    What do you think?

Emma:        This all sounds scary. It's like you're saying that avoiding marriage is a sign of health.

Therapist:    I don't think you necessarily need to break up to get a handle on your conflict. But I do think that your commitment conflict is unbalanced and that you each will have to give up something to save your relationship. Scott will probably need to give up his idealized view of his parents and acknowledge their critical and perfectionist behavior, self-centeredness, and withholding. He needs to consider dropping or modifying his idealization in some way that allows him to properly differentiate from his family of origin.

Emma:        Giving up my parents shouldn't be that hard.

Therapist:    It might be, if part of you continues to believe that you are unworthy of love. Never underestimate the power of an internalized conflict.

### Step 7. Alleviate commitment symptoms to develop a more durable relationship.

As the couple accepts their conflict and how each contributed to it, the couples therapist will notice an increase in mutual empathy. Symptoms may then begin to dissipate, even if the couple decide to end the relationship. And if it does end, the committed partner may no longer feel as if a soul mate has been lost, just someone who is conflicted about living being with them.

Emma:        You know Scott is not mean to me anymore. He seems to be accepting that the trap he is in is not completely my fault. I acknowledge that I pressure him, but I do less of it. I know now that I would be fighting for something that is not good for me. Scott should not want me out of obligation to his parents, and I need to allow myself to be wanted. Our sex life has not changed, but we talk more and argue less.

*Therapist:* What do you think Scott?

*Scott:* Emma's right. I feel sad that we both had to put ourselves through all this without even realizing it. I like Emma now more than ever. But it does seem like we need more work to decide what to do with our relationship. Whatever happens, at least we're finally dealing with it on a truthful, less combative level.

*Therapist:* That's right. Whatever you two decide will at the very least be true to the both of you.

Emma and Scott continued to work on their shared conflict and to treat each other with respect in the process, but they eventually decided to break up. Scott never wanted to marry Emma and neither partner could get past this issue. He had a hard enough time living with her. Nevertheless, there was very little drama in the split. Emma said that without therapy, their separation would have been a war filled with pain and bitterness. She said that the couple now get along like "good friends." Scott's parents refused to speak with Scott for approximately two months and even threatened to disinherit him. Eventually, however, they dropped the subject.

### Dontrell and Zendaya (See Figure 6.2)

Zendaya and Dontrell were a married Black couple in their early 30s. They had two young children together and a son from Dontrell's previous

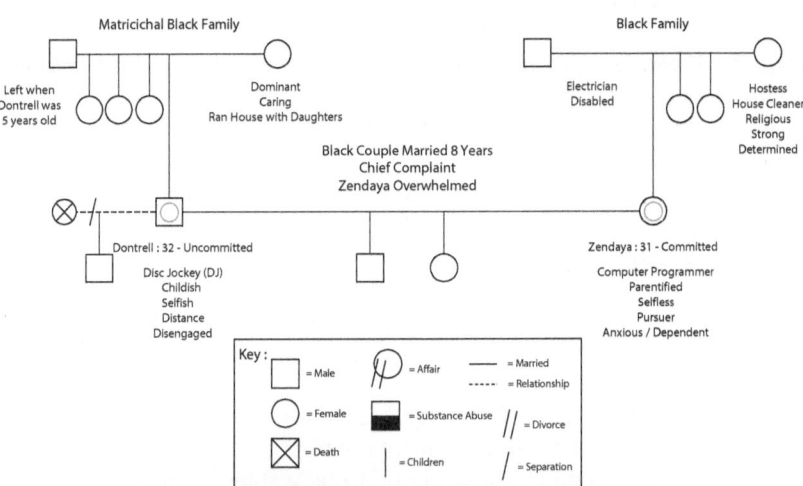

*Figure 6.2* Dontrell and Zendaya.

relationships. Zendaya was employed as a computer programmer at a large company. Dontrell was self-employed as a disc jockey (DJ).

### Initial Contact

Zendaya initially contacted me by email and followed with a telephone call. She said that she could not wait to see me. Along with her child-rearing duties, she held a full-time job and was the breadwinner of her family. Zendaya complained that her husband, Dontrell, spent more time with his friends than with his family. "He works at night, so why can't he watch our kids in the day? Why is it my mother's job?" Zendaya made it a point that she and her mother were also the primary caretakers of Dontrell's son from a now-deceased ex-girlfriend. The child was five years old when his mother died. When asked how Dontrell felt about therapy, Zendaya said he was indifferent but that he would "show up."

### First Session

Zendaya was angry with Dontrell. For most of the session, she scolded him on his "childish behavior." Dontrell, on the contrary, seemed to be tuning her out. When I asked him to comment, he dismissed her with a grunt and a wave of his hand. When he finally did speak, he said that she should "show him some respect and leave him be." He said he never promised her that he would be a model husband or father. This response frustrated Zendaya. Moving from anger she said she wasn't asking for perfection, just some help. She then pleaded with Dontrell to save her, but he was not empathetic. He said that raising a family was "women's work" and that Zendaya was trying to emasculate him. Zendaya's anger returned.

This appeared to be a transactional relationship. Dontrell needed someone to support him financially, care for his son, and meet his sexual needs. Zendaya met all these requirements and more. And she was right about his lack of commitment to her. Dontrell wasn't threatening to leave, but he was acting like a single man in marriage. He played the role of the uncommitted, and Zendaya played the role of the overwhelmed, committed partner.

### Genogram

Zendaya was the oldest of three sisters and the responsible one in her family. Her father was an electrician who fell off a scaffold and became permanently disabled when Zendaya was 10 years old. Her mother held two part-time jobs: one as a house cleaner and the other as a diner hostess. She described her mother as strong and determined. "My mother was very religious. And I think it was her faith that kept her going. I admire her."

Zendaya was tough and competent like her mother, and so she naturally fell into the parentified position. Her main job was to care for her younger sisters. And while they all remain close, Zendaya did admit they still call her "the general." The title is attributable to the days in which Zendaya ran the household with an iron fist.

Zendaya worked while in high school and saved enough money to attend community college. She then earned a scholarship to a small local university. While Zendaya had dreams of leaving home to attend an out-of-state college, she and her mother decided it would be best for her to stay close to home and commute so that she could continue to watch over the family. Zendaya studied computers and landed a job that paid well enough to support her mother and sisters. She said that she was proud of the fact that her career allowed her mother to work one part-time job, especially in her later years.

Although smart and attractive, Zendaya did not date in high school and throughout her life only had two relationships that lasted over a few months. She blamed this on the fact that she was far too busy to date. "My family was about surviving not playing," she said. The genogram gave no indication of sexual abuse or problems with substances in her family of origin. But the genogram did help me to see that Zendaya was more committed to her family than to herself.

Zendaya had no social life outside of family members. Even as an adult she socialized mostly with her sisters. Any of the couple's friends belonged to Dontrell, but Zendaya did not approve of these people. Zendaya was on blood pressure medication, which she attributed to her responsibilities.

Dontrell was the youngest child of four; he had three older sisters. Dontrell said that his father left when he was five years old, and he never saw him again. He said his mother and sisters do not mention his name. Dontrell grew up in a matriarchal household. His mother was in charge with the help of what he called her "three lieutenants." But he laughed when he said this and added that there were some benefits. He claimed that he was treated like a "prince" and that they made sure to meet his needs.

Dontrell also had talent in his own right. He was a star basketball player all through high school and gained a scholarship to a small college basketball power. He was not, however, strong in the classroom, and it took Dontrell five years to graduate. Dontrell's family was proud of him, but instead of becoming a lawyer, which they had hoped, he decided to follow his second passion: music. Once establishing himself as a DJ, Dontrell said that he fell in love with it and never looked back. Dontrell said that he was struggling with building his brand but that he saw a bright future.

Dontrell had many long-term relationships with women. He said that he only liked women who "had their heads on straight and didn't play games." But this seemed to be a projection because he admitted to cheating on most of them. Dontrell met Zendaya through a friend and knew instantly that she was a serious person. He called her the "whole package." Other than pot, he said that he takes no drugs or medications and only looks at porn when his friends do. He claimed that he was never abused in any way as a child or adult.

### Assessment Summary

Zendaya was parentified as a child and continues to caretake at the same level of intensity as she did when she was responsible for her mother and sisters. She takes care of her two children and her husband's child from a previous relationship. She also holds down a full-time job and could never accomplish all this without at least some help from her mother. But Zendaya is admittedly drowning in responsibility and desperately wants Dontrell to rescue her.

Ironically, Zendaya is not asking for an equal distribution of the domestic workload. She is, in fact, asking for very little, which fits with her parentified personality. She agrees that it is her job to take on all the responsibility even though she knows that it is killing her. She is only asking that her husband helps lighten her burden, but he is not committed enough to lend much of a hand. In fact, he adds more pressure to the situation by suggesting that the domestic and familial responsibilities should be solely the "women's job."

Dontrell was treated as if he was special by his mother and elder two sisters. He was free of any responsibility, and his family made sure of that. He might have been favored because he was the baby of the family or because he was the only male. Nevertheless, Dontrell was raised to let others take care of him. He committed to no one; even his family accepted his selfishness and expected nothing in return. His conflict, however, was that although he committed to no one, including Zendaya, he was ambitious and feared losing her. He said that he initially fell for his wife because he saw her as "all business." What he might have recognized is her ability to take care of business.

Zendaya was attracted to Dontrell's carefree attitude toward life, given her parentification. But she also disrespected his lack of commitment to her, the family, and his career. Consistent with her parentified pattern, she unconsciously took on Dontrell because of his potential to become another burden. Zendaya was the "all in" committed partner, selfless, loyal, and pursuing; Dontrell was the uncommitted spouse, selfish, disloyal, distancing, and disengaged. There was little intimacy in this relationship in part because it took on a parent–child dynamic. It was also a transactional relationship that was close to imploding. Zendaya could not continue to take sole responsibility for the family, and Dontrell is insulted that his wife insists that he contribute.

*Clinical Recommendations*

Dontrell must rescue his wife and demonstrate a commitment to his marriage and family rather than to himself and his friends. To do so, however, would mean that he would have to give up some of his princely benefits and negotiate a commitment that works for the marriage.

Zendaya will have to ask for what she deserves. And if Dontrell chooses to help, she must allow him to do the job without her taking over or micromanaging him. If he refuses, it might mean that he will never fully commit to her. If she cannot let him go, she is demonstrating that she doesn't deserve to be committed to.

*Treatment*

### Step 1. Determine the couple's interactional process or committed–uncommitted dynamic and how it enables the couple's symptoms in the context of attachment, love, intimacy, and passion.

It was relatively clear that Dontrell played the role of the uncommitted partner and Zendaya played the role of the committed partner. Zendaya pursued Dontrell to save her from her overwhelming responsibilities, but Dontrell resisted. He did not appear committed to the relationship other than in name. This committed–uncommitted dynamic impacted the couple's sex life. Zendaya had sex with Dontrell but showed little passion; like the couple's relationship, it was transactional. Love might be present, but Dontrell did not act as if he was in love with Zendaya. The couple also had very little, if any, emotional intimacy. The following vignette demonstrates how the couple's dynamic was exposed and its associated symptoms.

| | |
|---|---|
| *Therapist:* | Dontrell, it must be tough coming home to a worn-out, angry wife. Is she always after you for help? |
| *Dontrell:* | (Waves his hand as if to imply he doesn't really care). |
| *Therapist:* | Is that yes? |
| *Dontrell:* | Yeah. She's all over me all the time. She doesn't treat me like a man. |
| *Zendaya:* | I would if you acted like one and not some adolescent running around with his neighborhood homies… |
| *Dontrell:* | Housework is not my thing. It's women's work. |
| *Therapist:* | So, what is your job in the marriage, Dontrell? What is the job of a man? |
| *Dontrell:* | I work. And I'm trying to make it big so we can have everything we want. |

| Zendaya: | But I work too. And I make more money than you. So don't play that card with me. You just want to be taken care of. We made a commitment to each other in the church, and you're acting like that was nothing. |
| Dontrell: | It's not nothing. And I am committed. You don't see me going anywhere. |
| Zendaya: | I don't see you at all. |
| Therapist: | So, Zendaya, do you think the way the work is distributed in the marriage is unfair? |
| Zendaya: | That's what I've been saying. I'm in my 30s and I have high blood pressure. I don't want much, but I do need a little help. Having three kids is too much for a single parent, which is what I feel like. I'm the only one committed to this family. My kids all rely on me. They don't even ask their dad for much anymore. Thank God my mother helps me. But she's old and has some health issues. |
| Therapist: | Has this dynamic affected your attractiveness to Dontrell? |
| Zendaya: | We still have sex because I am still attracted to Dontrell, but I don't really enjoy it. I'm just trying to find anything that might bring Dontrell into the relationship with me. We don't speak anymore. We just make passing comments. There was a time we could talk. That's long gone. |

### Step 2. Expose the couple's internalized shared conflict with commitment and how each partner colludes in maintaining it.

| Zendaya: | If you're so unhappy, Dontrell, why don't you leave and find a more subservient woman? |
| Dontrell: | I never said I wanted to leave. I just want her to back off and treat me with more respect. |
| Therapist: | That's a noble request, Dontrell, but it doesn't seem like your behavior is helping your cause. In fact, it looks like you are making Zendaya angrier and more frustrated. Your behavior seems to make her respect you less. |
| Dontrell: | I act like this because of her. I don't want to leave. |
| Therapist: | I believe that you do not want to leave, Dontrell. But I also think you are checked out. You live with the family, but you're not sure how much of a commitment you want to make to them. It seems like there are two sides to you. |
| Dontrell: | What do you mean? |

*Zendaya:*    He means part of you is in the relationship and part of you is out of it.
*Therapist:*  And what about you, Zendaya?
*Zendaya:*    I guess I hate suffering like this. But I really haven't put my foot down over the years.
*Therapist:*  Yup. I know you're tough, but you have enabled Dontrell's behavior for a long time. That is why you are burned out. Perhaps you have done little but complain because you too have a conflict with commitment.
*Zendaya:*    How can that be? I feel as if I'm overly committed.
*Therapist:*  It makes sense that you chose Dontrell for a spouse and that you have been enabling him for a long time.
*Zendaya:*    Oh, so just because I married Dontrell that makes me guilty?
*Therapist:*  Not guilty but also a player in this conflict with commitment.
*Zendaya:*    Sounds more like bad judgment to me.
*Dontrell:*   Very funny. More disrespect.

### Step 3. Demonstrate how mate choice is based on this shared conflict.

Zendaya's last comment on her lack of judgment in choosing to marry Dontrell provided a good segue to show the couple how they unconsciously bonded over their conflict with commitment.

*Therapist:*  Zendaya, I was struck by your comment that you chose to marry Dontrell because of poor judgment. You may have been sarcastic, but I do think who we choose a partner to maintain our conflicts. For example, you have worked hard your entire life beginning as a child. If you truly believed that you deserved to be helped, wouldn't you have found someone who had no problem helping you? Wouldn't you have left if you felt that you truly deserved to be committed to? I am not saying you should divorce Dontrell. I am suggesting that you consider that your choice of partners may have been swayed by an unresolved conflict about getting your needs met.
*Zendaya:*    I get it. So, if it's like that, why did Dontrell choose me?
*Dontrell:*   Bad judgment also.
*Therapist:*  Dontrell is conflicted as well because he wants someone to take care of him but makes it so that they don't want to. He wants a home base and to be a man or respect, but he makes this difficult. You both have the same conflict with commitment.
*Zendaya:*    Why do we pick people who won't give us what we need?
*Therapist:*  That's an important question, and I think one of the keys to relationship problems. Let's try and answer it.

### Step 4. Broaden the couple's context beyond romantic commitment.

*Therapist:*  Zendaya, now that you have some idea of what your conflict might be, can you see it in other areas of your life?

*Zendaya:*  (Laughs). It is the story of my life. I have been caretaking for years. I just never realized there was a part of me that sabotaged getting the help I needed.

*Therapist:*  Is there anybody else on your back, Dontrell?

*Zendaya:*  Dontrell works on his own as a DJ because he's managed to get every employer that he's ever had angry with him. He has a reputation for being cool and aloof among his friends and family, but like me, his old bosses call it lazy and uninterested. Maybe now I can call it uncommitted.

*Dontrell:*  I don't want to be a slave to nobody.

*Zendaya:*  Slaves didn't make the money you and I make, Dontrell.

### Step 5. Expose the origin of each partner's conflict.

As noted, Zendaya was parentified in her family of origin. Her mother was a hardworking woman, but most of the day-to-day responsibilities fell on Zendaya. Without much reciprocity other than her mother's appreciation, Zendaya did not learn how to get her own needs met. As noted, this unconsciously has influenced the type of man she chooses to be with.

*Therapist:*  Zendaya, I want to follow up on your great question of where this conflict can come from. How might you have developed this kind of conflict?

*Zendaya:*  I guess I was raised to take care of everybody and to worry about them. You know, I've always fantasized about having an easy life, but I guess there's a part of me that would feel weird if I weren't involved in some project.

*Therapist:*  How about you, Dontrell?

*Dontrell:*  I don't know.

*Therapist:*  Can't you connect the way you were treated and the situation you are now faced with?

*Zendaya:*  Come on, Dontrell, admit it.

*Therapist:*  Don't help, Zendaya. You're off today.

*Zendaya:*  (Laughs) Right.

*Dontrell:*  I know what you're getting at. You think because my mother and sisters spoiled me, I want Zendaya to spoil me.

*Therapist:*  I do think they treated you as if you were "special" and required very little in return. And I also believe that this is the way you tend to view all relationships. That is, I think you do not feel as if you need to make much of a commitment, yet you expect others to commit to you unconditionally.

### Step 6. Differentiate from their respective families of origin to balance the shared conflict and to gain more control over it.

When a partner has received so much positive reinforcement over many years, it is especially hard for them to accept they will need any adjusting. In the following vignette, notice how Dontrell did not want to let go of his princely expectations and how Zendaya accepted that the parentified role did bring her control and prestige.

*Therapist:*   Dontrell, you were treated very well by your family. I suspect you're trying to replicate this in your marriage.
*Dontrell:*   I'd like the same respect I got from my family.
*Zendaya:*   But I'm not your mother or your sisters. I'm your wife.
*Dontrell:*   You're still a family member and a woman.
*Therapist:*   Dontrell, you do see that your wife is not going to accept the same role your mother and sisters played. Even though a part of her accepts it, she is clearly struggling.
*Dontrell:*   I know. But I can't make her happy. She'll always complain about something.
*Therapist:*   Maybe so, but you are making things worse. You want to be served. And if that's worth being tortured over for years to come, so be it. But if not, perhaps you could negotiate a compromise with Zendaya.
*Zendaya:*   I know I'm ready to stop acting like this parentified person. It's funny, now that you put a name on it, I see how crazy I've been.
*Therapist:*   Not crazy, just conflicted.
*Zendaya:*   Yes. It looks like both of us must give up our thrones.
*Therapist:*   Beautifully put, Zendaya. But easier said than done.

### Step 7. Alleviate commitment symptoms to develop a more durable relationship.

*Therapist:*   Dontrell, to make Zendaya respect you, you will have to pay a price: you will have to give up some of your princely ways. Notice I didn't say all of them – that will between you and Zendaya. But in return I believe you will be reciprocated.
*Dontrell:*   How?
*Therapist:*   Possibly better sex, less fighting, more respect, greater commitment, and you will be helping your wife to take better care of

|          |                                                                                      |
|----------|--------------------------------------------------------------------------------------|
|          | herself. Who knows, maybe it will extend her life. Doesn't that seem like a good deal? |
| *Dontrell:* | How do I know I'll get all that in return? I think I'll get complaints about something else. |
| *Zendaya:* | (Crying). I don't want to emasculate you, Dontrell. I just need your help. I can promise some of those things if you just be my husband. |
| *Dontrell:* | So, what are we talking about here? |
| *Zendaya:* | Hang out with the kids a little more. I'll do the food shopping and cleaning, but maybe spend a little more time at home with me. I'm not telling you to give up your friends. |
| *Therapist:* | Are you underestimating your needs, Zendaya? |
| *Zendaya:* | No, I'm being realistic. I know I tend to take control, and I also know Dontrell will never be completely rid of his prince thing. I can settle. |
| *Dontrell:* | Okay, I can try some of those things. |
| *Therapist:* | Good. As is, you have a failing business arrangement rather than a durable, committed relationship. And while a part of each of you is comfortable with this, another part is suffering greatly. |

I admit that I did not think this case had a positive prognosis. But Dontrell did as he agreed. He spent more time at home, freed Zendaya up by watching their children, and spent less time with his friends. And while he didn't give up all his princely ways, what he did offer earned him more respect from Zendaya and his children. He and his child from a previous relationship grew especially close.

Zendaya said she now feels like making love instead of meeting a requirement. As a result, there is more passion in their lives. The couple talk more, even though Zendaya still initiates most of the conversations. From a broader contextual perspective, Zendaya has been setting better limits with family and friends.

### William and James (See Figure 6.3)

William, a 42-year-old college professor, was partnered with James, a 31-year-old art teacher. The couple had been living together for approximately five years. They have no children.

#### Initial Contact

William made the initial contact for treatment. He complained that his partner James wanted to open their relationship to others and William hated

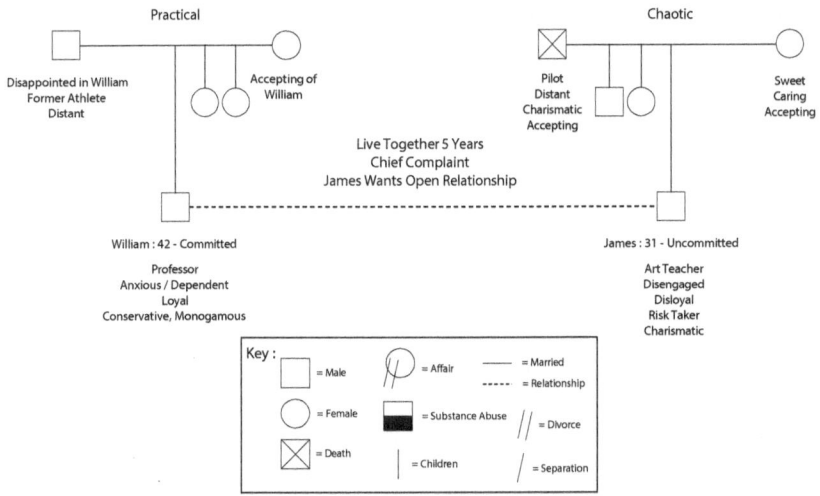

*Figure 6.3* William and James.

the idea. He feared doing so would ruin their relationship in part because he was not sure about James's commitment to him. According to William, James had a history of promiscuity and had cheated on him twice already. He also knew that James was not fulfilled by their sex life. However, he also believed that James was not satisfied with anything and was always looking for a new high. He said that although James would never admit to having any problems, he would attend couples sessions.

*First Session*

James and William were both very pleasant. However, it was no surprise that William was more anxious. He said that he knew James was upset about their sex life, but he didn't know what else to do. He said that he was open to experimenting sexually but knew that whatever he agreed to, James would eventually escalate it. He reiterated that opening their relationship was not an option for him.

James was laid-back and soft-spoken. It was as if he knew he had some power over William. He said that he was not intent on ruining the couple's relationship but that he was bored. As he spoke, I could see William deflate. He had an anxious, helpless expression. Rather than notice this, however, James continued to sell his idea. When I asked whether he was suggesting polyamory or swinging or some other alternative relationship, he said he was not interested in having another emotional relationship. He only wanted to be free to introduce new partners for sex.

William not only feared the deterioration of the relationship, but he also worried about catching a sexually transmitted disease (STD). James dismissed this by saying that William has obsessive compulsive disorder and thinks he will get a disease from everything he touches. He also said that William was still living in the 1980s (a reference to the HIV/AIDS crisis). When I pointed out that the odds of getting an STD does increase as the number of partners increases, James waved me off. He clearly did not like my comment because it failed to support his desire.

James said that he did not think he could stay in the relationship much longer unless something were to change. Apparently, he had been threatening to end the relationship off and on for some time over this matter. James argued that he was trying to improve the relationship by opening it, but William wasn't buying this. He reiterated that James is insatiable and has a history of being unfaithful to all his partners.

William knew of James's past, but he was taken by his good looks and charisma. He said that he has never been able to attract someone as handsome and popular as James. James smiled at hearing this, but I feared it only gave him more power to wield over William. William played the role of the committed, and James played the role of the uncommitted.

*Genogram*

William was the oldest of three children. From the time he was a young child, William was fascinated with the theater. He aspired to be a Broadway actor, but his parents thought it was too impractical and refused to support the idea financially. William did not put up much of a fight, but to his credit, he convinced his parents to fund a PhD in theater history, provided he, at least, be a college professor. William loved his career and was thankful his parents compromised.

William said that he "came out" when he was 14 years old and that his father was clearly disappointed. "I think he thought I could be a football player or something. I guess he wasn't paying attention," he said laughingly. William reported that his father probably never got over his announcement and still strains their relationship. "He's embarrassed to have a gay son. What can I say?" William's mother was much more accepting and was hurt by the distance created between William and the family because of her husband's stance. She missed the closeness she once had with William.

James is the youngest of three siblings. He described his childhood as somewhat chaotic given his father was an international airline pilot. James said his father was rarely home and that his family lived in many countries. He laughed when he said that all the moves cost him friendships, but he did learn to speak several languages.

Overall, James said that he did not have much to complain about. When his father was home, he got along great with him, and his mother was a "sweet and caring parent." He claimed that he loved both his parents. He described his father as a handsome, charismatic man whom he looked up to. But his father passed away from a heart attack when James was in his second year of college, and he wished that he had more time with him. He remained close to his mother and siblings.

James had lots of female and male partners over the years. He said that he came out when he was 15 years old and that his parents were very accepting. Because he was the baby of the family, everyone treated him "special," and he never even considered they would reject him. His transition to accepting himself as gay was relatively smooth.

James was very popular wherever he went. He was also a good athlete and so he said even the jocks liked him. James reported no abuse, and in his romantic relationships, he was always the one who ended them. He said, "Nobody has ever broken up with me."

Most of his relationships were short-lived prior to meeting William, but James did live with one man for five years. He said that he broke up with him because the man was obsessively jealous. James loved the attention and adoration but felt like a prisoner. He admitted that he has a history of cheating on his partners and could become bored quickly.

James did not take any drugs or prescription medication. He drank socially, and there was no history of substance abuse in his family of origin. He looked at porn, but he claimed he was not controlled by it. He said that his brother and sister have been married several times each, and he was always confused by this. He thought it may be that all the siblings have "a bit of wanderlust."

*Assessment Summary*

William and James were in a control struggle about opening their relationship. William, who played the role of the committed, loyal, anxious/dependent type, feared it would be the end of their union. He said that James, who played the role of the uncommitted selfish, distancing, disloyal type, could not be trusted, especially in such a sexually charged environment – he had a history of cheating and promiscuity.

William thought that James would never be satisfied and that his need to open their relationship was just another indication of his difficulty committing. William tried to please James, especially sexually. He even agreed to participate in some sexual acts that made him uncomfortable, but James was never-ending in his demands.

James believed that William was acting like a "scared and obsessive old man," still living in the past. He said he was bored with their relationship and that opening to others would help. He had William in a bind because he was a threat to cheat or leave if William did not succumb to his demands.

William was right in his assessment of James. I too believed that James was somewhat insatiable and quite capable of acting out sexually. Given James's history of family chaos and constant movement, it might be difficult for him to settle down without eventually feeling a need to move on. His childhood was chaotic, but it was also thrilling – and adventure waiting to happen. He met new people from different countries, immersed himself in different cultures, and learned to speak several languages. He was also popular wherever he went so he had no trouble adapting unlike many other children. But I also believed that James underestimated the many losses he suffered and that he longed for the structure that a man like William offered. This is, in part, why he entered a relationship with William to begin with.

William was somewhat conservative and a bit repressed. He was attracted to James's charisma and sense of freedom. He was also an older man who took pride in being in a relationship with such a handsome, popular man. Because William's friends were drawn to James, his social life dramatically improved.

William did not want to lose James. He felt that his life would be drab without him. However, James made him feel unsafe. He had already cheated, and I could tell that William had spent too much time worrying about what James would do next to threaten their relationship. In my opinion, the anxiety William was living with exhausted him. It was also affecting him physically (e.g., peptic ulcer, hair loss).

### Clinical Recommendations

James would have to grieve the losses from his childhood, especially his father's distance and death. His constant need for change may be a defense against these losses. If he can do this, however, he may come to believe that his need for a man like William is more important to him than he allows himself to acknowledge and feel.

William needed to build his self-esteem and self-worth rather than rely on someone like James to give him a life worth living. He has enabled James for too long and has suffered in the process. James now has him in a double bind, and the only way out is to strengthen himself and to allow James to leave if he must.

*Treatment*

### Step 1. Determine the couple's interactional process or committed–uncommitted dynamic and how it enables the couple's symptoms in the context of attachment, love, intimacy, and passion.

James played the role of the uncommitted partner, and William played the committed mate. James was bored with William, especially when it came to sex. As a result, James wanted to open their relationship. William objected, however. He would do just about anything for James except that. William believed that opening the relationship would be the beginning of the end in part, because James has a history of cheating and can be rather fickle.

The disagreement over opening the relationship caused turmoil, especially in the context of attachment: Is James suggesting an open relationship because he cannot attach to anyone? Does James really love William? Can James love? And did William feel he deserved to be loved?

| | |
|---|---|
| *Therapist:* | James, am I right in understanding that you might leave William if he refuses to comply with your wishes to open the relationship? |
| *James:* | I don't know. I just know that I'm not happy, and I don't think William alone can help me. |
| *William:* | I'll do just about anything except bring someone else into this. |
| *Therapist:* | But you also do not want to lose James. |
| *William:* | Right. I am in a bind. |
| *Therapist:* | James, do you see the bind William is referring to? |
| *James:* | Look, I know I have never done "commitment" well. But I am trying to rescue this relationship. I am losing my sexual passion for William, and I feel disconnected from him. |
| *Therapist:* | So, you're running low on commitment. |
| *James:* | Yeah. |
| *Therapist:* | How about you, William? |
| *William:* | I am dedicated to James, and he knows it. But he has become indifferent towards me. |
| *Therapist:* | His timer has run out. |
| *William:* | I never thought of it that way, but maybe so. |

### Step 2. Expose the couple's internalized shared conflict with commitment and how partners collude in maintaining it.

James's conflict with commitment was evident. He had a history of promiscuous behavior and has been in numerous relationships. Also, nobody has ever left James – he ended all his relationships. His history basically indicates that he may have a problem attaching, yet he keeps trying. William tolerates James's behavior and thus enables it. Given James' past and present behavior, it makes sense that William chose someone with the same conflict. The following vignette exposes this shared conflict and the couple's collusion to maintain it.

*Therapist:* William, when you first decided to become involved with James, did you consider his past?

*Wiiliam:* Yes. I was a little frightened. I worried whether I was going to be enough for him or just another statistic.

*Therapist:* Yet you went ahead with the relationship.

*William:* Yup. And here we are.

*Therapist:* But I suspect you were here before.

*William:* What do you mean?

*Therapist:* I thought James cheated on you in the past.

*William:* Oh right. Yes, he did. I caught him both times.

*Therapist:* And yet here you still sit.

*William:* I know. Sometimes I think I'm sicker than James.

*James:* (Laughing) I think you are.

*Therapist:* I don't think you are sick. But I do think you might have a conflict with allowing others to commit to you.

*William:* Well, that would make me and James a perfect pair.

### Step 3. Demonstrate how mate choice is based on this shared conflict.

*Therapist:* William, you said you and James are a "perfect pair." What did you mean by that?

*William:* Well, if James cannot commit and I cannot be committed to, we are a perfect match.

*Therapist:* What do you think, James?

*James:* Well, I know that I'm not great at committing, but I'm not sure why.

*Therapist:* We'll get to that. But do you agree with William that you two are a perfect match?

*James:* I guess. But it makes me feel bad. I mean, I don't want to contribute to his anxiety and low self-worth.

*William:* Believe me, you are.

*Therapist:* Feeling victimized, William?

*William:* Yes.

*Therapist:* But if you are in conflict, then part of you doesn't want to be committed too.

*William:* That's disturbing.

*Therapist:* Yes. But it makes sense that if you have a problem with others committing to you, and James cannot commit; you both share the same conflict. You probably even keep it alive.

### Step 4. Broaden the couple's context beyond commitment.

James already admitted that he had a history of commitment issues, so there was no need to waste time with this step. But I thought it was important to reinforce the pervasiveness of William's conflict because he saw himself as the primary victim in the couple dynamic.

| | |
|---|---|
| *Therapist:* | William, you seem like a very forgiving person. Are you generally like that? |
| *William:* | What do you mean? |
| *Therapist:* | Are you like this at work or with friends? |
| *James:* | He wants to know about all the people whom you let take advantage of you, William. |
| *William:* | I don't know. |
| *James:* | Oh, come on, William. Tell him about your nasty boss and how he humiliates you. William publishes quite a lot, but his chair always finds a way to make sure he doesn't get tenure. |
| *William:* | You don't know if he's the reason. |
| *Therapist:* | Well, who do you think is responsible? |
| *William:* | I don't know. But universities are not giving out tenure like they used to. |
| *Therapist:* | But how does he treat you? |
| *William:* | Well, not so nice. He rarely looks at me when he passes me in the hallway. |
| *James:* | Yeah. Maybe he's homophobic. |
| *William:* | I don't know. |
| *Therapist:* | How about your friends, William? Do they take advantage of you? |
| *James:* | Tell him about all the money you've lent to some of those deadbeat friends of yours. |
| *William:* | Well, that's true. My friends do take advantage of me, and I have a hard time setting limits with them. |
| *Therapist:* | The way you have with James. |
| *William:* | I guess so. Geez, I feel like an idiot. |
| *James:* | I saw that one coming. |

### Step 5. Expose the origin of each partner's conflict.

It was not difficult to locate the source of James's conflict with commitment. James came from a somewhat disorganized childhood with little attachment. His father traveled most of James's childhood and died relatively young. James loved and admired his father but always missed not having a relationship with him.

Another potential origin of conflict was the constant moving of his family because of his father's career. As soon as James got attached to anyone, he would lose them. James soon began to, at least on an unconscious level, fail to see the value in risking attachment. Again, he longed to connect and commit, and he tried it several times in his life, but he also did not trust it.

William's parents expressed disappointment in their son for being gay, especially his father. He wanted William to be an athlete, but William loved the theater. William desperately wanted to please his father and have a closer relationship with him. But his father could not accept William, and this manifested in William never feeling good enough. Thia led to conflict: William wanted to be accepted and to connect with others, but he was never sure whether he deserved to be committed to. The following vignette demonstrates how I helped each partner see the connection between their pasts and their present conflicts with commitment.

| | |
|---|---|
| *Therapist:* | James, there is something about you that puzzles me. You admit you've always had an attachment issue. But you seem as if you need a connection. You longed for a relationship with your father and for your parents' approval, and you value staying in contact with your two siblings. You can also form a romantic relationship even if they are short-lived. My point is you seem like two people: One who needs to make a commitment, and one who avoids it. |
| *James:* | I just think I'm an independent person. I really don't feel as if I really need someone. |
| *Therapist:* | Well, even if that's true, you do stay connected, and you continue to form relationships with other men. The issue is that you can only maintain a connection for a short time before you feel the need to escape. |
| *James:* | So, you're saying that I want to commit, and I don't want to commit at the same time. |
| *Therapist:* | Yes. Something like that. |
| *William:* | And I keep choosing people with a commitment conflict? |
| *Therapist:* | Right. That's how your conflict manifests. |
| *William:* | And all this comes from my past? |
| *Therapist:* | Is it that hard to believe? |
| *William:* | It's just hard to imagine my past having such a profound impact on my life today. |

## Step 6. Differentiate from their respective families of origin to balance the shared conflict and to gain more control over it.

| | |
|---|---|
| *Therapist:* | James, for you to gain more control over your problems with attachment and commitment, you will most likely have to risk further loss. |
| *James:* | (Laughs) I'm okay if I'm the one doing the breaking up. |

*Therapist:*   Right, no risk there. But to stay around long enough in a relationship and risk being abandoned scares you. Consider your
history with people and your distancing father. That's why I
suspect you must be in control of your relationships.

*James:*   I see that.

*Therapist:*   Okay, so it makes sense that you must hold the key to your
relationship with William in the palm of your hand. You are the
boss but only as long as William allows you to be.

*James:*   I never saw it that way.

*Therapist:*   And William, you will have to learn to get your needs met. You
must have experienced this before.

*William:*   Yes, and it felt good. But it didn't last.

*Therapist:*   That's because your conflict wouldn't allow it to. You will need
to get that under control to better manage your ability to connect and commit to James in a healthy way, or anybody for that
matter.

### Step 7. Alleviate commitment symptoms to develop a more durable relationship.

The aim here is to help James and William agree whether or not to open
their relationship to others. Armed with a better understanding of the influences their respective families of origin continue to have upon their relationships, they may be able to alleviate the symptoms of their shared
commitment conflict: James might be better able to commit and William to
insist that he do so.

*James:*   I can now see the influence my childhood has had on my ability to stay in a relationship, and it's hard to believe.

*William:*   I've always known I was a sucker for a pretty face, but I didn't
really know why. I just thought I was insecure.

*Therapist:*   You were, but not because of some deep flaw within you or
with your personality. Your conflict was in charge and compel-
ling you to get into relationships that do not offer you the love,
intimacy, and passion you claim to desire.

*William:*   I've been suffering my whole life, because of this conflict.

William and James were both very smart. Even though he was frightened,
William took the risk and told James that if he insisted on opening the relationship, he was going to end it completely. He said this in a sweet yet
firm way, not wanting to bully James. He told James that he did not wish to
pressure him any longer.

James surprised William and told him that his conflict had cost him many potentially good people and he no longer wanted to suffer any losses, even by his own hand. He admitted that if he could trust anybody not to abandon him it would be William – he agreed to take the concept of establishing an open relationship off the table. William said that there was always individual therapy, and James said that he may consider that.

## References

Betchen, S. (2022). *Couples in conflict: Clinical techniques for navigating sexual relationship control struggles.* Routledge.

Betchen, S. (2024). *Unmet expectations in couple and sex therapy: Helping couples negotiate realistic relationships.* Routledge.

Reese, R. J., Toland, M. D., Sloane, N. C., & Norsworthy, L. A. (2010). Effect of client feedback on couple psychotherapy outcomes. *Psychotherapy: Theory, Research, Practice,* Training, *47,* 616–630. https://doi.org/10.1037/a0021182

# The Therapist's Conflict with Commitment

# Chapter 7

# The Therapist's Commitment

I have found three types of commitment that the couples therapist will need in treating couples with commitment conflicts: (1) commitment to the profession; (2) commitment to the self; and (3) commitment to the couple being treated. Little to no commitment to the field may negatively impact the therapist's knowledge and skill base and, in turn, the efficacy of treatment. If the therapist is not committed to self-care, it may impact the physical and mental health of the therapist and, in turn, the therapist's ability to help the couple. And, if the therapist lacks commitment to the couple, they will most likely not improve, and the therapy may in fact do more harm than good. As described below, therapists may not be invested in all three types of commitment, but commitment to the couple is a necessity.

## Commitment to the Profession

Most of my mentors stressed the importance of maintaining a commitment to the field of marriage and family therapy throughout one's career. Some called it "making a contribution." By their definition, this meant keeping up with professional readings, conducting research or building theory through the publishing process, and presenting one's work, especially at professional conferences. One mentor also felt it was important to be active in professional organizations or on licensing boards. This stance reflected their values and what they tried to instill in me as a student. They truly believed that the more you study and immerse yourself in your craft, the more knowledge and skill you will gain, and the better chance you will have to achieve a positive, therapeutic outcome (Clay, 2019). A student once asked me if she should become a psychiatrist before training in couples therapy. I am not a psychiatrist, but my response was, anything that will add to your knowledge base and skill level will help. All this to say, anything that can add perspective should be welcomed.

DOI: 10.4324/9781003475743-11

## Commitment to the Self

Posluns and Gall (2020) wrote: "Stress, burnout, and professional impairment are prevalent among mental health professionals and can have a negative impact on their clinical work, whilst engagement in self-care can help promote therapist well-being" (p. 1). Maslach et al. (2001) defined burnout as a syndrome that consists of emotional exhaustion, depersonalization, and reduced feelings of accomplishment in one's work. Van Hoy and Rzeszutek (2022) found that burnout was correlated with age (younger therapists are more prone to burnout), gender (with mixed results), coping mechanisms and personality style (people who practice self-care are less effected by burnout), and work-related support systems (supervision). Studies have shown that therapists experiencing burnout cannot manage the therapeutic process and may put clients in danger (Berjot et al., 2013; Rupert & Morgan, 2005).

Eddington (2006) reported that the size of the caseload was a significant factor in the burnout of marriage and family therapists. I am always aghast when colleagues tell me they treat over 35 clients per week. A male colleague told me that for one year he saw an average of 45 couples per week. While he enjoyed the extra income, he said that it was not worth the depression he suffered because of it. Apparently, he had little time to do anything besides eat, sleep, and see clients, which contributed to a sense of alienation and isolation. He also spoke of the physical toll it took on his body. Once an avid exerciser, he had little time to visit the gym and soon suffered neck and back problems. He also found himself eating more fast food and adding a significant amount of weight.

The term "compassion fatigue" was originally applied by Joinson (1992) to the nursing profession but is now used commonly to describe therapists who have difficulty nurturing because of clinical burnout and suffering (Paiva-Salisbury & Schwanz, 2022). Figley (1995) applied the concept to those helpers who suffered from secondary posttraumatic stress disorder. According to the Substance Abuse and Mental Health Services Administration (2024), some of the symptoms of compassion fatigue are feeling tired and overwhelmed, angry, frustrated, and cynical. Physical effects may include headaches, heart palpitations, and insomnia.

Therapists, many of whom were parentified in childhood (Brown, 2014), are especially vulnerable. They are far better at considering the needs of others at the expense of their own and are more vulnerable to enmeshed therapeutic relationships (Begni, 2005). Jung (1946/1966), in the context of psychoanalysis, referred to these caretaking clinicians as "wounded healers." The following brief example is not of a burned out or emotionally fatigued therapist but a parentified child who, as a couples therapist, had difficulty setting limits with couples, creating great stress for herself.

A colleague, I'll refer to as Ellie, failed to charge a fee for service that was commensurate with her level of education and experience. She also neglected to send out bills and was uncomfortable collecting her fees. Ellie claimed that she was fine with her style of practice, that is until her mortgage payment came due, or her car needed expensive repairs. Then she would panic and attempt to borrow from friends and family. After one scare I could not help but ask her: "How can you live like this? It would probably kill me." She then confessed that she felt too guilty to charge clients for treatment, especially those struggling financially. She spoke of her childhood parentification and how she never took the time to take care of herself. "I never thought of myself," she said. "My parents and siblings were so needy and demanding." Ellie admitted that she was committed to meeting her own families' needs and equally committed to the needs of her clients. Ellie told me that she hadn't had a vacation in years. I didn't think she could afford one anyway.

Without a commitment to the self, first and foremost, it will be hard to commit to the profession and to competently commit to one's caseload over the span of a career. A talented colleague, Mandy, unfortunately chose to leave the field because of burnout and compassion fatigue rather than learn to practice self-care. She decided that she could not afford personal therapy, and the clinic she worked at demanded that she carry a large caseload without adequate supervision. Add to this her long commute to work and her vast administrative duties.

A caretaker from childhood, Mandy was still looking after her disabled mother, and her personality made it difficult for her to separate her work from her personal life. That is, she suffered from insomnia and chronic gastrointestinal problems. While I tried to support her as best I could, she was set on pursuing what she felt was a less demanding profession. I believe the field lost a potentially excellent marriage and family therapist.

## Commitment to the Couple

According to the American Association for Marriage and Family Therapy (2015) *Code of Ethics*: "Marriage and family therapists do not abandon or neglect clients in treatment without making arrangements for the continuation of treatment." Abramson (2022) found that terminating treatment without making allowances for a client can exacerbate the client's symptoms. To manage this process appropriately, the author strongly recommends a sufficient termination process and suggests some good reasons for ending a course of treatment: (1) if the therapist cannot adequately treat the client's needs; (2) the client is not benefitting from the treatment; (3) the therapist becomes involved in an inappropriate relationship with the client; and (4) the client threatens or assaults the therapist.

The implication here is when the therapist agrees to accept a couple into treatment, he/she is making a commitment to the couple that should not be broken without good reason. Even then, the couple should be clinically provided for *via* an appropriate and skillful transfer or termination. In supervising both experienced and therapists and trainees, I have identified the following reasons for lack of commitment to the couple:

**Anger** – Some couples therapists may be angry with their clients for a variety of reasons, including not responding quickly enough in treatment. I received a referral from a cognitive behavioral therapist who was angry and frustrated because a couple he saw was resistant to doing homework assignments. Rather than process his own angry feelings toward the couple in a productive manner (Berthoud & Noyer, 2020) and address the couple's resistance, he referred the couple to me.

In the first session the couple demonstrated what Schwartz et al. (2021) described as "hostile resistance." They said they felt abandoned by the initial therapist and took it out on me. Once this dynamic was processed, the couple adjusted and did quite well.

**Overwhelmed** – Doherty (2002) claimed one of the mistakes an inexperienced therapist can make is to give up on a couple because the therapist feels overwhelmed. Some couples present with many symptoms, confusing the therapist and giving the impression they have too many insurmountable problems for the therapist to handle. I have found that if the couples therapist focuses on the presenting symptoms or context only, he/she can become easily deflated and want to refer the couple to someone they perceive has more ability to treat such cases.

**Dislike** – Therapists are human and will not like every couple. When a trainee admits they dislike a couple, I first recommend that they look for something in each partner that they can empathize with. If therapists can see beyond the couple's defensive structure, they may discover something familiar, like their own issues with intimacy (Tartakovsky, 2017). If this fails, I usually instruct the trainee to find something they like about the couple. And if this does not work, I recommend that the trainee look for something they respect.

A trainee suggested that she might refer a couple to me who had questionable ethics and had hurt many people in their lives. The trainee said that she had to get rid of them because they "disgusted her." She thought both partners were sociopathic. As supervision continued, the trainee gave me several examples to support her view of the couple, but it was clear that they were also highly intelligent and very well educated. Rather than refer the couple, I recommend that she try to connect with them based on a certain admiration for their intelligence and business acumen. She was able to do this long enough to better understand that their ruthlessness in business emanated from an underlying shame they both experienced growing up poor.

It is quite common for a couples therapist to like one partner and not the other. Partners often present differently but are alike in the way that binds them. Therefore, if one partner is unethical the other might be as well or at the very least enables the other. A colleague new to couples therapy referred a couple to me because she said that she "could not stand" the husband. She did not believe a word he said, and although he admitted to having had an affair, the therapist did not believe it was his first or would be his last. If the therapist would have done a bit more digging rather than lose her objectivity in the wake of the wife's victimization, she might have learned what I did: that the wife had an affair many years before and that the husband never knew about it.

*Countertransference* – The concept of countertransference is not routinely applied in the marriage and family therapy literature (Furgal et al., 2013), but many therapists find it impossible to avoid and potentially useful (Solomon & Siegel, 1997). A trainee I was supervising just had a miscarriage, and the couple she was seeing had just had a baby. The trainee told me that although she felt bad having to refer the couple, she had to because she could not handle the case emotionally. She claimed that she was still working through her anger and grief. The couple was shocked by the quick referral. They liked the therapist, but she needed to explain that the timing of the events made working with them too difficult for her.

Another trainee insisted that I allow him to refer a couple to a sex therapist because the husband was into kink. As a sex therapy supervisor, I told the trainee that I could have helped him with the case. But he said that he "didn't want to talk about it." He also made it clear that he did not want to treat any sex therapy cases because of a history of sexual abuse. I recommended personal therapy, but he said he was already getting help.

And a colleague told me that she was going to transfer a couple because she "hated" the husband. She told me that if there ever was a client whom she wanted to "punch in the face," it was him. I asked her how he was able to get her so angry. She admitted he reminds her of her hypercritical father, questioning every intervention or point she made.

*Fear* – According to Pope and Tabachnick (1993), most of the professional literature on "therapist fear" focuses on the fear of assaults. It specifically examines the risk rather than actual patient attacks. Most therapists cannot commit to a client they are physically afraid of even if working through it might benefit the client greatly.

A colleague transferred a male client, Mark, to me because he stood up in a couples session and told her that she was "ruining" his life. The therapist said that she felt physically threatened and kicked Mark out of her office. She later referred him to me. After meeting with Mark, I found that he had a history of being abandoned. His own mother has not spoken to him in years.

Mark's dynamic was to annoy someone to the point that they leave him, and the therapist had fed into the same pathological dynamic by kicking Mark out of treatment. Mark tried the same thing with me using the session fee as his hammer. He pestered me relentlessly to give him receipts when he knew that I gave them out at the end of each month. But rather than kick him out of treatment, I said to him: "You can continue to try to get me to abandon you, but I won't do it. You're not going to get me to kick you out just like all the other people have in your life. You're stuck with me." Mark eventually accepted monthly receipts.

I was away on vacation when one of my trainees called the police on the husband of a couple. He apparently requested an individual session and showed the trainee an unloaded gun he had hidden in his jacket. The therapist got scared and alerted the clinic, who, in turn, called the police and had him arrested. Knowing the case well, I reminded her that on more than one occasion I told her that this man had a crush on her, but she found it too disturbing to process. I told her that if she had listened, her client may not have been compelled to show her his "big gun."

Besides safety concerns, two other common fears are a client's suicide and a fear of being sued (Pope & Tabachnick, 1993). With reference to suicide, I have known colleagues who were so anxious about a client doing self-harm that they referred the client elsewhere. While it may be appropriate to engage a psychiatrist in the matter or to seek supervision, a premature referral to another therapist could feed into the client's self-deprecating feelings, especially if they are suicidal because of prior abandonment.

**Hopelessness** – Sometimes you can continue to treat a couple but give up on them while still in process. I have treated many couples over the years who for some reason never put an ounce of effort into their treatment, and I surmised never would. It is hard for the therapist to commit to those who are not committed to themselves or the treatment process.

The wife of a couple I treated verbally tortured her husband almost every day. But even after a year of treatment, it was apparent he was not able to do what it would take to stop her, such as threatening to leave the relationship. Even when I tried to support him, both partners would gang up against me. When I told the couple that I think they were wasting time and money in couples therapy, and that individual treatment would be more appropriate, they chose to stay in treatment with me. I felt bored, somewhat defeated, and could not help but lack commitment to them.

**Conflict of Interest** – A therapist should not establish a relationship with a couple when there is a conflict of interest. This is one of the most problematic issues faced by therapists and one of the most common ethical violations reported (Anderson, 2011; Rollins & Grames, 2021). But sometimes a couples therapist only learns of this conflict in the middle of treatment. For example, the husband of a couple told me that his wife was having an affair with another client of mine. I had no idea this was happening and decided to transfer all parties to other therapists. While the husband agreed with my decision, his wife and her lover were upset and claimed they were feeling abandoned. They wanted me to continue treatment with all of them because I knew everyone involved.

**Conflict of Values** – Some couples therapists are not open to treating problems that conflict with their values, be it in a religious or a moral context. A colleague enraged a female client because she refused to treat her. Apparently, the client was having an affair with a married man and was seeking sex therapy to help her function better sexually with her lover. The therapist thought the client's request was offensive, deceitful, and pathological.

In 2023, the Supreme Court ruled in favor of a Christian Evangelical web designer who refused to design a website for a same-sex couple about to wed. This example begs the question: Must therapists commit to every couple who requests treatment? At least part of the answer can be found in one's professional code of ethics. The following codes are that of marriage and family therapists and social workers, respectively.

**American Association for Mariage and Family Therapy Code of Ethics (2015) – 1.1 Non-Discrimination:**

Marriage and family therapists provide professional assistance to persons without discrimination on the basis of race, age, ethnicity, socioeconomic status, disability, gender, health status, religion, national origin, sexual orientation, gender identity, or relationship status.

**National Association of Social Workers Code of Ethics (2021) – 4.02 Discrimination:**

Social workers should not practice, condone, facilitate, or collaborate with any form of discrimination on the basis of race, ethnicity, national origin, color, sex, sexual orientation, gender identity or expression, age, marital status, political belief, religion, immigration status, or mental or physical ability.

But what about the rights of therapists? Barsky (2024) addressed this dilemma and called for mental health providers to seek supervision, consultation, and educational and professional programs to help them to separate their personal and professional values . He believed that transferring unwanted cases could do harm to clients, making them feel rejected or abandoned. Barsky takes a hard line against discrimination in the treatment setting and is clearly in tune with both codes presented.

In sum, to have a successful, durable relationship, partners must be committed to each other, to the relationship, and to the treatment process. But it will also take the dedication of a competent couples therapist who is skillful in technique, knowledgeable in clinical theory, and adept at self-care and limit-setting. The therapist must have the ability to join with a couple and follow-through with treatment in most cases.

## References

Abramson, A. (2022). When therapy comes to an end. *Monitor on Psychology, 53*, 80. https://www.apa.org/monitor/2022/07/career-therapy-conclusion

American Association for Mariage and Family Therapy (AAMFT). (2015). *Code of Ethics*. https://www.aamft.org/Legal_Ethics/Code_of_Ethics.aspx

Anderson, S. K. (2011). Professional boundaries and conflict of interest: Providing benefit and avoiding harm. In K. S. Kitchener & S. K. Anderson (Eds.), *Foundations of ethical practice, research, and teaching in psychology and counseling* (2nd ed.). (pp. 209–244). Routledge.

Barsky, A. E. (2024, January). Are therapists required to serve every client? Free expression and the law about denying service to potential clients. *Psychology Today*. https://www.psychologytoday.com/us/blog/agens-scientiam/202401/are-therapists-required-to-serve-every-client

Begni, I. (2005). *Therapists: From family to clients* [Unpublished doctoral dissertation]. University of Wolverhampton.

Berjot, S., Altintas, E., Lesage, F., & Grebot, E. (2013). The impact of work stressors on identity threats and perceived stress an exploration of sources of difficulty at work among French psychologists. *SAGE Open, 3*, 1–11. https://doi.org/10.1177/2158244013505292

Berthoud, L, & Noyer, T. (2020). Therapist anger: From being a therapeutic barrier to becoming a resource in the development of congruence. *Person-Centered and Experiential Psychotherapies, 20*, 34–47. https://doi.org/10.1080/14779757.2020.1796771

Brown, F. (2014). Psychology career motivation: Were you a parentified child? Michigan School of Psychology. https://msp.edu/psychology-career-motivation-parentified-child/

Clay, R. A. (2019). Running start...to a great career: Keeping up with the research. *American Psychological Association*. https://www.apaservices.org/practice/business/ecp-column/keeping-up-research

Doherty, W. J. (2002, November/December). Bad couples therapy. *Psychotherapy Networker*, 26–33.

Eddington, C. A. (2006). *Burnout in marriage and family therapists* [Master thesis, Utah State University]. All Graduate Theses and Dissertations. https://digitalcommons.usu.edu/etd/2561

Figley, C. R. (Ed.). (1995). *Compassion fatigue: Coping with secondary traumatic stress disorder in those who treat the traumatized*. Brunner/Mazel.

Furgal, M., Janus, B., & Bobrzynski, J. (2013). On the possibility of using countertransference in couples therapy. *Psychoterapia, 165*, 29–44. https://www.researchgate.net/publication/290655386_On_the_possibility_of_using_countertransference_in_couples_therapy

Joinson, C. (1992). Coping with compassion fatigue. *Nursing, 22*, 116, 118–119.

Jung, C. (1946/1966). The practice of psychotherapy Essays on the psychology of transference and other subjects. Fundamental question of psychotherapy. In H. Read, M. Fordham, G. Adler, & W. McGuire (Eds.), R.F.C. Hull (Trans.), *The collected works of C. G. Jung* (2nd ed., Vol. 16, pp. 163–240). Princeton University Press.

Maslach, C., Schaufeli, W., & Leiter, M. (2001). Job burnout. *Annual Review of Psychology*, *52*, 397–422. https://doi.org/10.1146/annurev.psych.52.1.397

National Association of Social Workers (NASW). (2021). *Code of Ethics*. https://www.socialworkers.org/about/ethics/code-of-ethics

Paiva-Salisbury, M. L., & Schwanz, K. A. (2022). Building compassion fatigue resilience: Awareness, prevention, and intervention for pre-professionals and current practitioners. *Journal of Health Services Psychology*, *48*, 39–46. https://doi.org/10.1007/s42843-022-00054-9

Pope, K. S., & Tabachnick, B. G., (1993). Therapists' anger, hate, fear, and sexual feelings: National survey of therapist responses, client characteristics, critical events, formal complaints, and training. *Professional Psychology Research and Practice*, *24*, 142–152. https://doi.org/10.1037/0735–7028.24.2.142

Posluns, K., & Gall, T. L. (2020). Dear mental health practitioners, take care of yourselves: A literature review on self-care. *International Journal for the Advancement of Counseling*, *42*, 1–20. https://doi.org/10.1007/s10447-019-09382-w

Rollins, P., & Grames, H. (2021). Sanctioned licensing board violations for marriage and family therapists spanning a 10-year period. *Journal of Marriage & Family Therapy*, *48*, 641–642. https://doi.org/10.1111/jmft.12523.

Rupert, P. A., & Morgan, D. J. (2005). Work setting and burnout among professional psychologists. *Professional Psychology: Research and Practice*, *36*, 544–550. https://doi.org/10.1037/0735–7028.36.5.544.

Schwartz, R. A., Chambless, D. L., Mirod, B., & Barber, J. P. (2021). Patient, therapist, and relational antecedents of hostile resistance in cognitive-behavioral therapy for panic disorder: A qualitative investigation. *Psychotherapy*, *58*, 230–241. https://doi.org/10.1037/pst0000308

Solomon, M. F., & Siegel, J. P. (Eds.). (1997). *Countertransference in couples therapy*. Norton.

Substance Abuse and Mental Health Services Administration (SAMSHA). (2024). Compassion fatigue and self-care for crisis counselors. https://www.samhsa.gov/dtac/ccp-toolkit/self-care-for-crisis-counselors

Tartakovsky, M. (2017). Therapists spill: When I dislike a client. *PsychCentral*. https://psychcentral.com/lib/therapists-spill-when-i-dislike-a-client#1

Van Hoy, A., & Rzeszutek, M. (2022). Burnout and psychological wellbeing among psychotherapists: A systemic review. *Frontiers in Psychology*, *13*. https://doi.org/10.3389/fpsyg.2022.928191

# Epilogue

The future of marriage as we know it is in question, as made evident by the steady decline in marriage rates. Brown et al. (2020) claimed that over a 25-year period, the marriage rate for women ages 18–49 dropped from 72% to just 57%. And according to data collected in 2021 by the U.S. Census Bureau, the marriage rate in the United States was down from 16.3 to 14.9 per 1,000 women (Washington & Anderson, 2023). As of 2022, there were approximately 48.78 million men and 42.69 women who never married (Korhonen, 2023). According to the World Economic Forum, the key reason for this decline is a lack of eligible or "marriageable" men as defined by: (1) men with poor economic standing and (2) men who are unavailable because of incarceration (Gould-Werth, 2018). This does not necessarily account for those highly educated women who are deferring marriage to pursue careers (Betrand, 2016).

The decline in Black marriages in the United States is perhaps most startling. According to data collected by the U.S. Census Bureau, in 1970, 35.6% of Black men and 27.7% of Black women were never married. In 2020, however, marriage rates dropped precipitously with 51.4% of Black men and 47.5% of Black women who never married (Washington & Walker, 2022). Scholars have attributed this drop-off to racial inequities leading to declining employment for Blacks, the rising incarceration rates of Black men, a smaller pool of Black men for Black women to marry, and lower educational opportunities and achievement leading to economic constraints on Blacks (Raley et al., 2015).

Despite the dour statistics, people continue to form relationships. But there is a significant rise in sexual experimentation (Singal, 2016). Many, for example, are rejecting traditional monogamy in favor of alternative relationship styles. Approximately 3–7% of the population claim to routinely engage in consensual non-monogamy, with 20% having tried it (Scoates & Campbell, 2022). And Monto and Neuweiler (2023) reported an increase in people reporting sex with both men and women. These findings are supported by my clinical practice, where I have seen a dramatic increase in the

DOI: 10.4324/9781003475743-12

number of non-traditional relationships over the past 10–15 years and not just among young people. It is not uncommon for a 50-year-old couple to present for treatment with issues related to their polyamorous relationship or because of struggles with their swinging lifestyle.

Craig and his wife, Heather, agreed to practice polyamory but sought treatment because Craig thought that his wife was spending more time with her partner than with him. While he was not suggesting the couple return to a monogamous lifestyle, he did want Heather to be more committed to their relationship.

Ben and Diana were swingers who had been in the lifestyle for many years without any significant problems. Ben insisted on treatment, however, because Diana had recently broken two rules the couple agreed upon before becoming swingers: (1) no sex with others in the family home and (2) no more than two sexual encounters with the same individual – they believed this rule might help prevent either spouse from falling in love with someone else. What the couple did not account for, however, was the power of Diana's need for risky public displays of sex or exhibitionistic behavior; something that embarrassed Ben. It seems that when she found a man with the voyeuristic tendencies, she lost control and could not stop herself from having sex with him several times in the family home and in several public locations.

With the advent of the Internet, it is now easy to use pornography to make up for any sexual deprivation in a relationship (Hesse & Floyd, 2019), and many couples are taking advantage of this. Lawrence claimed that he was addicted to oral and anal sex and yet he married a woman, Eve, who was not fond of either. Even when Eve did perform one of these acts, it was solely to please Lawrence – she did not especially enjoy it and was void of passion. Lawrence sought treatment because he looked to the oral and anal sex in porn to stimulate him and it was putting his marriage in jeopardy. He also came to realize that he was using porn as a weapon against his wife for what he perceived as her withholding behavior toward him.

Fred and Terry were practitioners of bondage, discipline, domination, submission, sadism, and masochism (BDSM) primarily for Fred's enjoyment and stimulation. Terry said that she never especially liked the activity, but she did admit that Fred was better aroused when it was included in their lovemaking.

Both partners agreed to treatment but with different agendas. Terry wanted Fred to give up BDSM, and Fred wanted her to continue it. The real crisis broke, however, when Terry refused to participate anymore. In response, Fred found a woman on the Internet who would engage in kink of any kind. Both Fred and Terry were angry with each other, but Terry considered Fred's response adulterous and was threatening to end the relationship if he refused to stop seeing the other woman. Fred reluctantly ended his relationship but would not give up on trying to convince Terry to re-participate in the BDSM.

With the changes happening in relationship dynamics, and the ever-increasing ability to substitute whatever is perceived missing in one's relationship with someone or something else, couples and therapists alike will have to adjust their definition of romantic commitment. It stands to reason that when more people or opportunities are added to a couple's life, commitment becomes even more difficult to maintain. How can partners in a polyamorous relationship operationalize their commitment in a way that would be satisfactory to all participants? And with so many outlets available to satisfy oneself, why would one individual even consider committing solely to another?

I would argue that it is important for couples to acknowledge the importance of romantic commitment in sustaining a lifelong relationship, no matter the lifestyle. And that couples should pay close attention to all the ingredients of commitment (e.g., attachment, love, intimacy, and passion) and take immediate action if one or more is missing or lacking enough to leave a partner dissatisfied.

I also believe that intimacy is especially vital in this environment. Mitchell (2003) was right in urging partners to risk expressing their true needs and desires to one another. He believed that couples mistakenly refrain from doing so for fear of upsetting the stability of their relationship, only to do so in the end. Ignoring relationship problems, as many couples do, might have a better chance of ending a relationship than in previous generations. In this sense, assessing and treating romantic commitment are, now more than ever, critical to a couple's relationship and ensuring that it is built to last.

## References

Betrand, M. (2016). Highly educated women are less likely to get married, aren't they? *World Economic Forum.* https://www.weforum.org/stories/2016/06/highly-educated-women-are-less-likely-to-get-married-arent-they/

Brown, S. L., Lin, I.-F., & Mellancamp, K. A. (2020). The rising midlife first marriage rate in the U.S. *Journal of Marriage and Family, 84,* 1220–1223. https://doi.org/10.1111/jomf.12861

Gould-Werth, A. (2018). Marriages in the US are on the decline. Here's why. *World Economic Forum.* https://www.weforum.org/stories/2018/11/what-upticks-in-u-s-economic-inequality-andincarceration-mean-for-marriage//

Hesse, C., & Floyd, K. (2019). Affection substitution: The effect pornography consumption on close relationships. *Journal of Social and Personal Relationships, 36,* 3887–3907. https://doi.org/10.1177/0265407519841719

Korhonen, V. (2023). Marital status of the U.S. population 2022, by sex. *Statista.* https://www.statista.com/statistics/242030/marital-status-of-the-us-population-by-sex/

Mitchell, S. A. (2003). *Can love last? The fate of romance over time*. Norton.

Monto, M. A., & Neuweiler, S. (2023). The rise of bisexuality: U.S. representative data show an increase over time in bisexual identity and persons reporting sex with both women and men. *The Journal of Sex Research, 61*, 1–14, https://doi.org/10.1080/00224499.2023.2225176

Raley, R. K., Sweeney, M. M., & Wondra, W. (2015). The growing racial and ethnic divide in U.S. marriage patterns. *Future Child, 25*, 89–109. https://doi.org/10.1353/foc.2015.0014

Scoats, R., & Campbell, C. (2022). What do we know about consensual non-monogamy. *Science Digest, 48*, 1–5.

Singal, J. (2016). Americans are sexually experimenting way more than they used to. *Huffington Post*. https://www.huffpost.com/entry/americans-are-sexually-ex_b_10285024

Washington, C., & Anderson, L. (2023). Is your state in step with the national marriage and divorce trends? National marriage and divorce rates declined from 2011 to 2021. U.S. *Census Bureau*. https://www.census.gov/library/stories/2023/07/marriage-divorce-rates.html

Washington, C., & Walker, L. (2022). Marriage prevalence for Black adults varies by state. District of Columbia had lowest percentage of married black adults in 2015–2019. *Census Bureau*. https://www.census.gov/library/stories/2022/07/marriage-prevalence-for-black-adults-varies-by-state.html

# Index

Note: *Italic* page numbers refer to figures.